THE DENTAL BURNOUT SOLUTION

Also by Dr. Sharon Grossman

The Burnout Solution: 7 Steps from Exhausted to Extraordinary

Don't Buy Their Lunch, Buy Their Loyalty: The Daily Habits That Actually Retain Employees

Motivated to Stay: 100 Strategies for Keeping Your Best People

The Stress Advantage: Lessons from the Tennis Court

Wheely Good Team Building: A Roller Skating Retreat to Revive a Company

The Currents of Change: How to Thrive During Corporate Transitions

The Zen of Work: Transforming the Tension in Your Brain, Body, and Business

All books are available at www.amazon.com/author/sharongrossman

THE DENTAL BURNOUT SOLUTION

Building a Practice You Love
Without Losing Yourself

Dr. Sharon Grossman & Dr. Kalli Hale

First Edition: 2026

For permission requests, contact the publisher at:
Warrior Publishing, LLC
drsharongrossman.com/contact

ISBN: 978-1-952437-07-6

Disclaimer

The information in this book is intended for educational purposes only and does not constitute professional psychological, medical, or legal advice. Readers are encouraged to seek qualified professional support for individual concerns.

Praise For The Dental Burnout Solution

"Ambition, drive, and a machine-like work ethic are virtues—until they aren't. Left unchecked and without guard rails, they hit a point on the curve where virtue becomes vice and breakdown is inevitable. *The Dental Burnout Solution* is Dr. Kalli Hale's gift to a profession running on fumes.

Part warning, part example, this book is a tale of two paths with two vastly different destinies. One, chosen by default, leads straight to a high-volume, anxiety-driven breakdown. The other is forged deliberately. As a nationally renowned mentor, clinician and leader in airway health, Kalli has built a complete framework for longevity by turning the exact, five-stage systemic diagnostic tools she uses on her patients back onto her own life. The results are profound, and the process is clear. Dr. Kalli Hale is an alchemist, and this book is the golden extract of her sacrifice, suffering, and triumph. She is a gift to the profession, and this is her gift to us."

— **Alastair MacDonald**, TEDx Speaker, Private Strategic Advisor, and Founder of the Sovereign Dentist Mastermind

"*The Dental Burnout Solution* is a timely, honest, and practical roadmap for every dentist who has ever felt trapped by the profession they once loved. Dr. Kalli Hale and Dr. Sharon Grossman do more than describe burnout. They show dentists how to rebuild their practices, protect their health, and create a career that can actually last."

— **Howard Farran, DDS, MBA**, Founder of Dentaltown

"Every dentist I coach has felt the slow erosion this book names so honestly… and almost none of them were ever handed a way out that respected how we actually think and work. Grossman and Hale didn't write another self-help book—they built a system for practicing dentistry without losing yourself, and it's the rare resource I'd put in the hands of every doctor and owner I'm blessed to lead and coach."

— **Dr. Jason Tanoory**, Founder of Finger Lakes Dental Care & Host of the *Dental Lighthouse Podcast*

"Burnout has become one of the greatest challenges facing dentistry today, and Dr. Kalli tackles it with honesty, wisdom, and practical solutions that actually work. This book is a gift to our profession and a must-read for any dentist who wants to build a sustainable, fulfilling career without sacrificing their health, relationships, or sense of purpose."

— **Dr. Mark Costes,** Founder of the Dental Success Network & Author of *Pillars of Dental Success*

Contents

Preface

This book did not start as a collaboration. It started as a search for relief. Dentistry is such a unique profession. You're expected to be the best clinician, all while running a business (something you get no training for in dental school). Hiring, firing, payroll, crown margins, perio charting, equipment purchases, google reviews, continuing education, audits…all of that.

Dr. Kalli Hale was burned out. Not the kind of tired that goes away after a long weekend, but the kind that sits in your chest, hijacks your sleep, and makes you wonder how something you once loved became so heavy. Dentistry had not failed her overnight. It had worn her down slowly, quietly, and efficiently—like enamel under constant acid attack.

Like most dentists, her path looked predictable and impressive from the outside. Dental school. Freedom. Debt. Long hours. High expectations. Expected to know everything. The unspoken agreement that if you are smart, capable, and disciplined enough, you will be fine. Everyone else seems to be pushing through [keywords: seems to be…], so you assume this is just what success costs.

Dentistry can be incredibly lonely if you don't have help, a mentor, or a friend you feel safe to admit failure to. The mental toll of dentistry creates a unique burnout style and desperation for escape. Thus, the slow boil.

Patients were messaging Dr. Kalli on Facebook at night. She was friending people she barely knew because saying no felt uncomfortable. She'd be answering Zoom whitening questions at 8 p.m. while her kids played nearby. She told herself it was temporary. She assured herself she could handle it. She thought that once things settled down, she would breathe again.They never did.

By the time the foundation gave way, it did not look like weakness. It looked like productivity and professionalism layered over constant anxiety. It looked like checking the schedule at night and rehearsing worst-case scenarios. It looked like a blood pressure reading of 186 over 120 during a normal conversation—her body screaming what her mind refused to acknowledge. It looked like standing in the parking lot, hand on her car door, seriously considering driving away and never coming back.

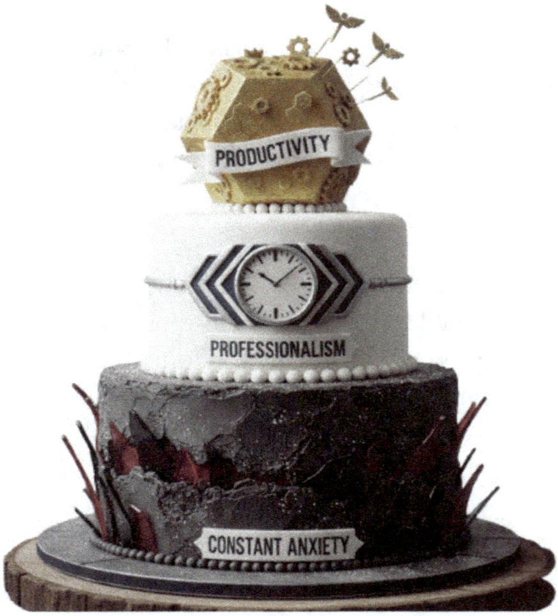

At that point, Dr. Kalli did what many dentists do quietly and alone. She started googling self-help & burnout books, hoping to find something—anything—that could help her make sense of what was happening and, more importantly, help her stop it.

That search led her to Dr. Sharon Grossman's work. That search changed her life.

Dr. Sharon Grossman started her career as a psychologist doing therapy the traditional way. She saw patient after patient, day after day, listening deeply, holding emotional weight, and showing up fully for people in crisis. The work was meaningful, but she was acutely aware of the risk. She knew that caring professions burn people out when there are no systems in place to protect the person doing the caring. Rather than wait for burnout to happen to her, she built a system to prevent it.

She began researching why highly capable, conscientious professionals break down despite doing "everything right." Over time, clear patterns emerged. The same personality traits showed up again and again: perfectionism, difficulty delegating, inability to say no, catastrophic "what if" thinking. The same cognitive traps. The same physiological warning signs ignored until the body forced a shutdown. The same slow erosion that people mistake for normal stress until it becomes something much more dangerous.

That research became her book, *The Burnout Solution.* This book incorporated the most successful lessons and mindset shifts she was teaching her therapy clients, which evolved into a framework. It became a mission to help people understand that burnout is not a personal failure or a character flaw. It is a predictable outcome when high responsibility meets flawed systems, unrelenting standards, and a nervous system that never gets to reset.

Dr. Kalli did not just read Dr. Sharon's book. She worked it. She applied it in real time, in the operatory, under pressure. She took notes with a highlighter in hand. She did the exercises between patients. The tools did not ask her to quit dentistry or care less about her patients. They helped her think differently, regulate her nervous system, recognize her "what if" spirals before they hijacked her day, and make decisions that actually reduced the load she was carrying instead of adding to it.

When she finally reached out, the email was simple and unfiltered:

"Dr. Grossman,

I am truly one of your biggest fans. Your book, The Burnout Solution, changed my life.

I hope I get the chance to tell you about it one day.

Dr. Kalli Hale"

That email started a conversation. That conversation made something obvious very quickly. General burnout advice is good, but specifics about how burnout shows up for dentists is even better. Here's why:

You work in someone's mouth—one of the most vulnerable, anxiety-inducing spaces on the human body. You make hundreds of micro-decisions a day that matter clinically, financially, and legally. You manage pain, fear, finances, time pressure, staff dynamics, insurance limitations, and your own perfectionism—all while performing physical labor that requires cognitive precision and emotional regulation at the same time. Then you go home and replay the day in your head, wondering if you made the right treatment decisions, if that patient will leave a one-star review, if you should have even said yes to that case.

Most burnout books do not account for that reality. They talk about self-care without addressing the operatory. They talk about mindset without touching practice systems. They offer inspiration when what dentists need is immediate, practical relief. They assume you can meditate your way out of a schedule that has you double-booked with no bathroom break until 2 p.m.

When Dr. Sharon heard Dr. Kalli's story—and when Dr. Kalli described how these psychological tools played out in a real dental practice with real patients, real staff conflicts, and real financial pressure—the conclusion was obvious.

Dentistry needed its own burnout book.

One grounded in psychology and tested in the chair. One that respected how dentists think, how they work, and how much responsibility they carry. One that did not patronize them with generic wellness advice but instead gave them a framework that actually fit their lives.

That is what this book is.

The Dental Care Pathway: A Framework That Fits How Dentists Already Think

We built this book the way you would approach a complex dental case. You do not start with cosmetics. You do not whiten before you treat decay. You follow a proven clinical pathway: You diagnose the problem, stability the damage, restore what's been lost, fortify to prevent future breakdown, and scale by expanding capacity sustainably.

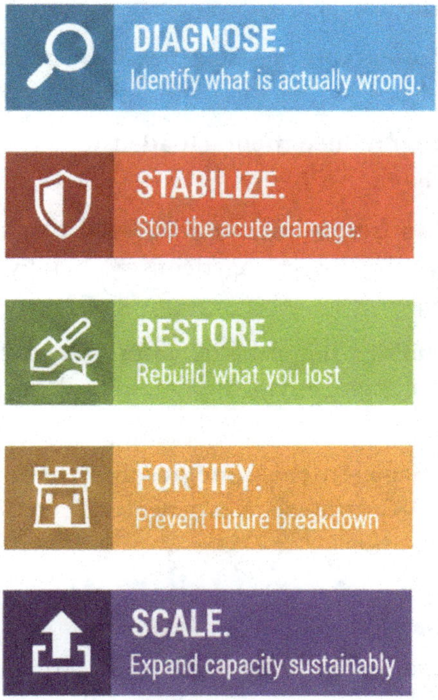
DIAGNOSE.
Identify what is actually wrong.
STABILIZE.
Stop the acute damage.
RESTORE.
Rebuild what you lost
FORTIFY.
Prevent future breakdown
SCALE.
Expand capacity sustainably

Burnout recovery works the same way. You cannot skip steps. You cannot "push through" inflammation and expect a stable result. You have to treat the root cause, not just the symptoms.

This book follows that pathway. It blends the science of burnout recovery with the realities of dental practice. It respects how dentists think, how they work, and how much they carry. It does not ask you to love dentistry unconditionally or walk away from it dramatically. It shows you how to practice in a way that does not cost you your health, your relationships, or yourself.

What You Will Find Here

There is no hustle worship in these pages. There is no guilt for feeling exhausted. There is no advice that assumes you can simply *want* your way out of burnout or that a bubble bath will fix a systemic problem.

What you will find instead:

- **Practical tools you can use between patients.** Not someday. Today.
- **Systems that reduce mental load** instead of adding more tasks to your already-impossible list.
- **Real stories from someone who lived this** and rebuilt from the inside out—not by leaving dentistry, but by changing how she practiced it.
- **The psychology behind why you think and react the way you do** under pressure, and how to interrupt those patterns before they drain you.
- **Practice management strategies** that prevent burnout instead of creating it—from patient experience design to staff training to schedule control.

Dr. Kalli is a dentist who burned out. Although at one time she wanted to walk away from dentistry, she didn't. Instead, she found a way to recover by changing how she *thought* about it. That recovery became the foundation for something she never thought possible in the height of her distress. Multiple practices. New models of care. Leadership roles. A life designed intentionally, not survived reactively.

None of that happened because she worked harder in the chair. It happened because she realized her mindset was limiting her and her current mode of practicing was not sustainable long term.

The Core Message

Here is what we need you to understand before you turn another page.

You can fix this. But your mind needs the refresh button.

You are not failing. But your body will fail if you don't fix YOU..

You are not a bad dentist. But dentistry will burn you out if you don't create boundaries.

The system you were trained in—the one that prioritizes productivity over sustainability, that equates boundary-setting with weakness, that never once taught you how to run a business or manage your nervous system—never prepared you for *longevity*.

It trained you to fix teeth, not to thrive in practice for 30+ years.

This book shows you how to build what was never given to you: a sustainable model for practicing dentistry without sacrificing everything else that matters.

You spent years learning how to save teeth.

Now it is time to learn how to save yourself.

Dr. Sharon Grossman & Dr. Kalli Hale

How to Get the Most From This Book

Throughout this book, you'll find bonus tools, worksheets, assessments, and implementation resources available at:

www.dentalburnoutsolution.com

Download them as you go and use them to put these concepts into practice immediately.

PART I
Diagnosis

CHAPTER 1

Micro-Erosion: How Dentists Burn Out Without Noticing

Have you ever looked at your schedule and wondered when the day stopped belonging to you?

Have you ever told yourself "it's just one message," "just one emergency," "just one more case," and then realized those tiny concessions have taken over your life?

Have you ever felt the edge of your patience thinning. Not because you're weak. Because the accumulation of small asks, small deadlines, small interruptions, has been grinding you down without your permission?

Most dentists don't burn out with a dramatic collapse. There's no cinematic breaking point. It's quieter than that. More deceptive. It looks like micro-erosion. The slow wear of daily compromises that feel reasonable in the moment. Until they aren't.

Maybe it started with answering a patient's message at night. It felt kind. You were being helpful. Then suddenly you're fielding a steady flow of after-hours questions while your family is in the next room.

Maybe you stayed late for one emergency. Then another. Then it became routine, and your "compassion" turned into a pattern you couldn't undo.

Maybe you said yes to a case you didn't have time for, because saying no felt uncomfortable. Then you looked at your schedule one day and realized you had no open space, no margin, and no control. You just kept moving from room to room, hoping nothing went sideways because you had zero bandwidth if it did.

Have you ever been so deep in accommodation that you couldn't see a way out?

That's micro-erosion. The little things that don't feel dangerous until they've rewritten how you practice and how you live.

You ignore the physical signs because "this is just dentistry." The elevated blood pressure. The chest tightness. The sleep that never refreshes you. You brush off the spiraling thoughts about patient outcomes, staff friction, and finances because it all feels normal. Everyone else seems to push through it, right?

But somewhere along the way, the job stops being something you do. It becomes something that owns you. Your schedule leads. Your phone interrupts. Your decisions shrink to what other people need instead of what keeps you healthy, centered, and capable.

Have you ever stepped into the operatory already braced for the worst? Not because anything bad happened, but because the erosion has been happening so long you've forgotten what ease feels like? Or your assistant said the patient was upset?

If any of this sounds familiar, you're not permanently broken. You're not "bad at boundaries." You're not a failure. You're experiencing what happens when micro-erosions go untreated. And the good news. Once you recognize the pattern, you can change the trajectory.

This chapter shows you how to spot the early fractures—and more importantly, how to stop the slow decay before it collapses.

The Slow Creep

Burnout is not a light switch. It is not something that flips from "fine" to "broken" overnight.

It is a spectrum. A continuum. A slow creep from manageable stress to chronic overwhelm to complete depletion.

Most dentists live somewhere in the middle of that spectrum for years without realizing it. They know they are tired. They know they are stressed. They know something feels off. But they assume this is just what it costs to run a practice, raise a family, and pay off six figures of student loans. After all, everything leading up to becoming a dentist made this level of stress oddly familiar.

They tell themselves:

- "Everyone else seems fine, so I should be too."
- "You asked for this, you chose to become a provider. This is the price you pay."
- "This is just a busy season. It'll calm down soon."
- "I'm fine. I just need a vacation."

But here is what most people do not understand about burnout.

It is not the same thing as being *tired*.

Yes, exhaustion is part of it. But burnout is a specific syndrome with distinct components that go far beyond needing more sleep.

The Burnout Triad: More Than Just Exhaustion

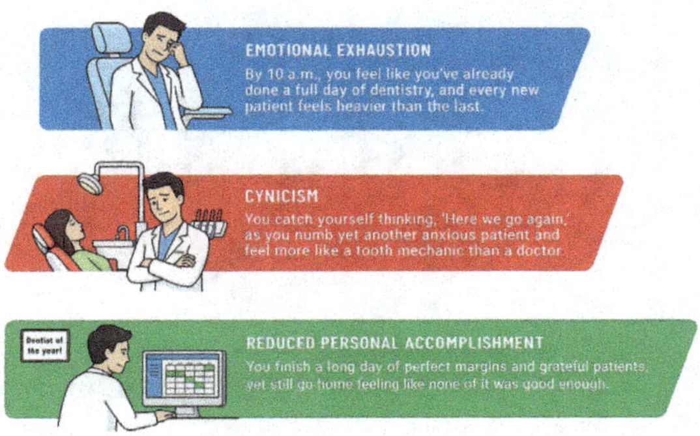

The World Health Organization defines burnout using three core dimensions:

1. Emotional Exhaustion (Mental Fatigue)

This is the component most people recognize. It is the bone-deep tiredness that does not go away after a weekend. It is waking up already drained. It is feeling like you have nothing left to give by 10 a.m. It is the sense that your internal battery is dead and no amount of rest seems to recharge it.

For dentists, this often shows up as:

- Difficulty concentrating during procedures
- Forgetfulness (missing details you would normally catch)
- Irritability with patients or staff over minor issues
- Physical symptoms: headaches, muscle tension, digestive problems, insomnia
- Emotional numbness or feeling like you are running on autopilot

Dr. Kalli remembers the moment she knew something was seriously wrong. She was sitting in the operatory having a normal conversation with her associate dentist when a wave of dizziness hit her. Not from standing up too fast. Not from low blood sugar. Just sitting. Talking.

Her assistant took her blood pressure.

186 over 120.

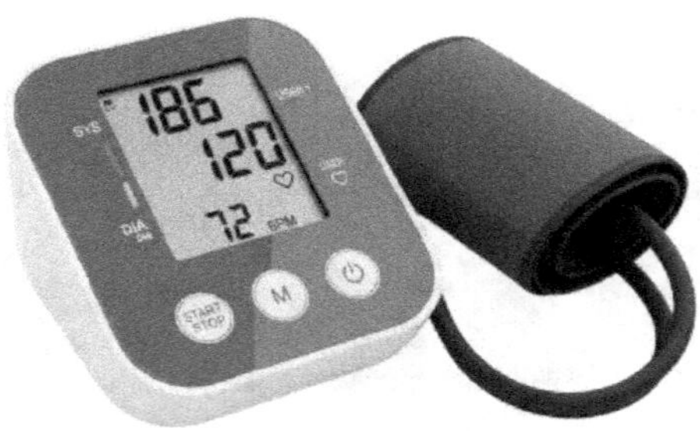

Crisis-level hypertension. In the middle of a workday. During a calm moment. Her body was screaming what her mind refused to acknowledge: *You are not fine. This is not sustainable. Something has to change.*

2. Cynicism (Depersonalization / Mental Distancing)

This is the component most dentists do not see coming—and the one that feels the most disturbing when it arrives.

Cynicism in burnout is not about having a bad attitude. It is a protective mechanism your brain uses when it is overwhelmed. You start to emotionally distance yourself from the people you are supposed to care about.

Patients stop being people and start being problems to solve.

Staff members stop being teammates and start being obstacles in your way.

The work you once loved starts feeling meaningless.

You catch yourself thinking:

- "I don't care if they're happy with the crown. I did it right."
- "If they don't want treatment, fine. I'm not going to beg them."
- "Why am I even doing this? No one appreciates it anyway."

This is not you being a bad person. This is your nervous system trying to protect you from emotional overload by shutting down your capacity to care.

Dr. Kalli describes this phase with brutal honesty: "I started to lose my empathy for the practice. I was starting to lose my care for what the experience was like for people when they walked in my doors—something that I had curated so carefully for so long."

When you stop caring about the thing you built, when patient outcomes feel irrelevant, when you are just going through the motions—that is not apathy. That is burnout.

3. Reduced Personal Accomplishment (Inefficacy)

The third component is the one that breaks people.

You start to feel like you are bad at your job. Like you cannot do it effectively anymore. Like no matter how hard you try, it is not good enough.

Even when objective evidence says otherwise—your outcomes are fine, your patients are happy, your practice is thriving—you feel like a fraud. Like you are failing. Like you used to be good at this and now you are just barely surviving. Get me off this merry-go-round.

For high-achieving dentists, this is devastating.

You spent years becoming excellent. You worked harder than most people can imagine. You sacrificed your twenties to get here. And now the thing you worked so hard to master feels impossible to do well.

You start doubting yourself:

- "Did I miss something in that exam?"
- "Should I have done that differently?"
- "Am I even cut out for this anymore?"

The irony? Most burned-out dentists are still performing at a high level. Their clinical work is solid. Their patients trust them. But they *feel* incompetent because their internal measuring stick has become impossible to reach.

The Human Function Curve: Finding "The Hump"

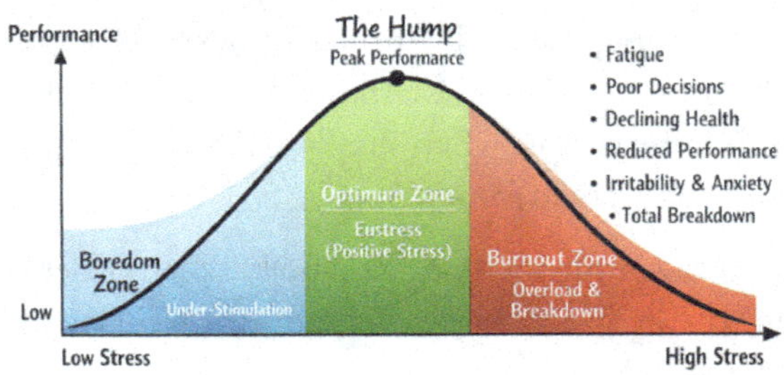

There is a concept in psychology called the **Human Function Curve**, and it explains why so many capable, hard-working dentists end up burned out despite doing everything "right."

Here is how it works.

At low levels of stress, you are under-stimulated, bored, not challenged enough. Performance is okay, but you are not firing on all cylinders.

As stress increases, performance improves. You get sharper, more focused, more efficient. This is the zone where you feel engaged, capable, and productive. This is where most dentists live during their first few years in practice. The work is challenging, but it feels good. You are learning, growing, building something.

This phase is often called "eustress"—positive stress that motivates you.

But here is the problem.

There is a peak.

A point on the curve where stress stops helping and starts hurting. Where additional pressure no longer makes you better—it makes you worse.

This is **"The Hump."**

Beyond The Hump, more stress leads to:

- Fatigue
- Poor decision-making
- Declining health
- Reduced performance
- Irritability and emotional volatility
- Eventually, total breakdown

Most dentists do not realize they have crossed The Hump until they are already in decline. They keep pushing because pushing always worked before. They assume that if they just work a little harder, stay a little later, see a few more patients, things will get better.

They do not.

Because once you are past The Hump, **more effort produces worse results.**

Dr. Kalli lived this. She was producing over a million dollars a year in airway cases. From the outside, she looked wildly successful. But internally? She was barely holding it together. Every new patient was no longer a victory; they were a burden. Every clinical decision felt like a lead weight. She was sprinting toward an exit ramp, ready to abandon a decade of building because she couldn't find the "leak."

She thought the problem was dentistry. She was wrong. The profession was just the stage where her burnout was performing—the actual "why" had almost nothing to do with the drill.

And because she was a high achiever—because she had always been able to push through—she kept going. She ignored the warning signs. The elevated blood pressure. The sleepless nights. The racing heart. The constant anxiety.

Until her body forced her to stop.

Why High Achievers Miss the Warning Signs

Here is the cruel irony of burnout.

The people most at risk are often the ones least likely to see it coming.

Why?

Because the traits that make you an excellent dentist—perfectionism, high responsibility, relentless work ethic, commitment to your patients—are the same traits that blind you to burnout until it is severe.

You are trained to push through discomfort. Dental school taught you that. Residency reinforced it. Your entire career has rewarded you for ignoring your own needs in service of the work.

So when burnout starts creeping in, you do what you have always done.

You push harder.

You tell yourself:

- "I can handle this."
- "Other people have it worse."
- "I just need to get through this busy season."
- "I'm fine. I'm just tired."
- "I have to make payroll."

And because you *have* handled hard things before, because you *did* survive dental school and boards and building a practice, you assume you will handle this too.

But burnout is different.

It is not a challenge you can outwork. It is a signal that the system itself is unsustainable.

Dr. Kalli's parents told her she was burned out. Her husband told her she was burned out. Her body was telling her she was burned out.

But she did not believe it. Or maybe she did not want to believe it. Because if she was burned out, that meant something was deeply wrong. And she did not have time to deal with something deeply wrong.

So she kept going. Until the day she ran out the back door of her office, contemplating leaving a full day of patients (and her team) to figure it out themselves.

That is when she finally admitted it.

I cannot do this anymore. I won't do this anymore. This has to be fixable because I am way too good at being a dentist.

Self-Assessment: Where Are You on the Spectrum?

Before we go further, you need to know where you are.

Burnout is not binary. It is not "burned out" or "fine." It is a spectrum, and your position on that spectrum determines what you need to do next.

Answer these questions honestly. Not how you think you *should* answer them. Not how you want to appear to others. How you *actually* feel right now:

Emotional Exhaustion

- Do you wake up already dreading the day ahead?
- Do you feel drained by the end of most workdays?
- Do you struggle to concentrate during procedures?
- Do you find yourself irritable or short-tempered with patients or staff?
- Do you feel emotionally numb or like you are just going through the motions?
- Do you have physical symptoms (headaches, tension, digestive issues, insomnia) that seem tied to work stress?

Cynicism / Depersonalization

- Do you find yourself caring less about patient outcomes than you used to?

- Do you feel mentally distant from your patients during appointments?
- Do you catch yourself thinking negatively about patients or staff?
- Do you feel like the work you do does not really matter?
- Have you started to resent your practice or the demands it places on you?
- Do you feel like patients or staff are just problems to manage rather than people to serve?

Reduced Personal Accomplishment

- Do you doubt your clinical skills even when outcomes are good?
- Do you feel like you are not as effective as you used to be?
- Do you question whether you are cut out for dentistry?
- Do you feel like a fraud or impostor despite your credentials and experience?
- Do you feel like nothing you do is good enough?
- Have you lost the sense of satisfaction you used to get from your work?

If you answered yes to 2-3 items in one category: You are in the early stages. This is the time to intervene before it progresses.

If you answered yes to 4+ items in one category or yes to items across all three categories: You are in moderate to severe burnout. You need immediate stabilization strategies (which we will cover in Chapter 4).

If you answered yes to most or all of these questions: You are in crisis. This is not sustainable, and your health is at serious risk. You need help now—whether that is a coach, a therapist, or a trusted mentor who can help you create an emergency plan.

Bonus Resource

Download a printable version of the Dental Burnout Spectrum Self-Assessment at:

www.dentalburnoutsolution.com

Use it as a quarterly check-in, share it with colleagues, or have your team complete it during staff development discussions.

The Truth No One Tells You

Here is what you need to understand before we move forward.

No matter how bad things feel right now, how burned out you might be, how cynical or ineffective you might find yourself, this is not about shame.

Burnout is a predictable outcome when high demands meet limited resources, unrelenting standards, and a system that was never designed for sustainability.

You were trained to fix teeth. You were not trained to manage a business, lead a team, regulate your nervous system under pressure, or design a practice that supports your wellbeing. And while none of that is your fault, it *is* your responsibility to change it. Your health and career depend on it.

Why? Because no one else is coming to fix this for you. Not your staff. Not your patients. Not the insurance companies. Not the dental associations. This is on you.

And the good news—the part that makes this entire book worth reading—is that you *can* change it. Dr. Kalli did. And if she can go from standing outside ready to quit to running 10+ thriving practices while picking her kids up from school every day, you can too.

But first, you have to stop believing the lie that burnout is the price of success.

It is not.

It is the price of an unsustainable system.

And in the next chapter, we are going to examine exactly what you bring to that system—the personality traits, thinking patterns, and unconscious beliefs that make dentists uniquely vulnerable to burning out.

Because once you understand *why* you are burning out, you can start to do something about it.

CHAPTER 2

THE TYPE A TRAP: What You Bring To The Chair

Dr. Kalli Hale thought she was organized. She thought she was responsible. She thought she was doing what dentists are supposed to do—care deeply, work hard, and hold herself to the highest possible standards.

What she did not realize was that the same traits that made her an excellent dentist were also driving her straight into burnout.

High school: straight A's, sacrificing social life to maintain her GPA because anything less than perfect had consequences.

College: pre-dental track, every exam feeling like it determined whether she would get into dental school. Organic chemistry finals that kept her up at night, convinced that one bad grade would ruin everything.

Dental school: the proving ground. Eighty-eight students started. Six did not make it to graduation. She watched classmates she respected struggle and eventually leave, and she thought, *How could you get this far and not finish?* She did not understand yet how the pressure accumulates. How the relentless demand to perform without support breaks even the strongest people.

Then she graduated. She thought the hard part was over. It was not.

Because the personality she had built to survive high school, college, and dental school—the one that equated achievement with worth, that could not tolerate mistakes, that said yes to everything and no to almost nothing—did not suddenly change when she started practicing.

She brought it with her into the operatory, into her business, into every patient interaction and staff meeting and scheduling decision.

And it nearly destroyed her.

The Personality Profile of Burned-Out Dentists

If you lined up a room full of burned-out dentists and asked them to describe themselves, you would hear the same words over and over:

- Perfectionist
- Overachiever
- Responsible
- Conscientious
- Hard-working
- Detail-oriented
- Self-critical
- Driven

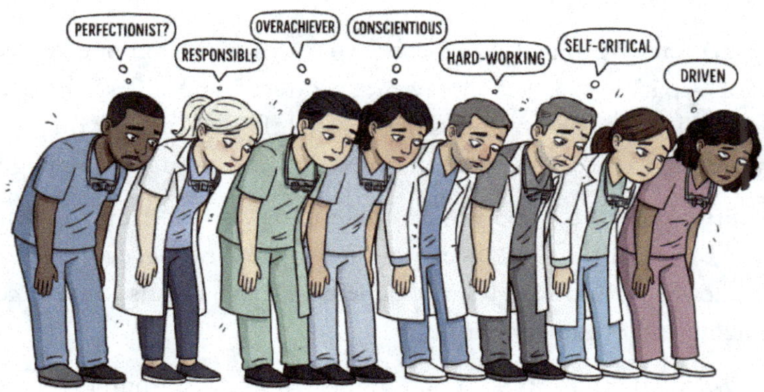

These are not bad traits. In fact, they are often the traits that make someone an excellent clinician.

But they are also the traits that, when taken to an extreme, create a perfect storm for burnout.

Research on burnout consistently shows that certain personality characteristics make people more vulnerable. In a comprehensive study published in the *Journal of Applied Psychology*, researchers Swider and Zimmerman (2010) found through meta-analysis that personality traits significantly predict burnout outcomes, with some traits increasing vulnerability while others provide protection.

High conscientiousness. You feel deeply responsible for outcomes. You do not cut corners. You follow through. You take ownership. This makes you reliable and trustworthy. It also means you carry the weight of every patient, every case, every decision—even the ones outside your control.

Perfectionism. You have high standards for yourself and your work. You notice details others miss. You are not satisfied with "good enough." This drives excellence. It also means you are never satisfied, never done, never able to rest because there is always something that could be better. Research by Hill and Curran (2016) in *Personality and Social Psychology Review* found that perfectionism has increased substantially among college students over recent decades, with socially prescribed perfectionism (believing others expect perfection from you) showing the steepest rise—and this dimension is particularly linked to burnout.

External locus of control. You believe your worth is determined by external validation—patient satisfaction, reviews, production numbers, approval from colleagues. This makes you highly motivated. It also means you are at the mercy of things you cannot control, constantly chasing a moving target.

Difficulty saying no. You want to help. You do not want to disappoint people. You assume that if you just try harder, you can meet everyone's needs. This makes you compassionate and generous. It also means you overcommit, overextend, and eventually burn out.

Anxiety-driven thinking. Your mind is always running scenarios, anticipating problems, preparing for worst-case outcomes. This makes you prepared and proactive. It also means you live in a constant state of low-grade stress, always bracing for disaster.

Sound familiar?

If you are reading this book, chances are you recognize yourself in at least three of those descriptions. Maybe all of them.

Here is what you need to understand: **These traits are not flaws. But they become liabilities when there are no systems in place to protect you from yourself.**

The Triangular Trap: How Perfectionism Keeps You Stuck

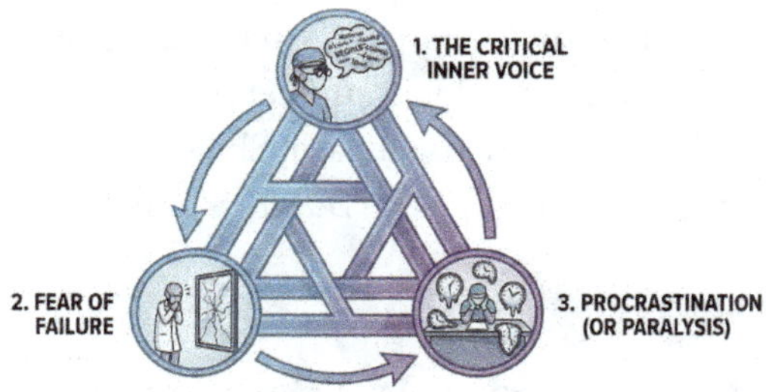

Perfectionism is not about doing excellent work. Perfectionism is about believing that your worth depends on flawless performance.

And for dentists, this creates a vicious cycle that psychologists call the **Perfectionistic Trap** or the **Triangular Trap.**

It has three components that feed each other:

1. The Critical Inner Voice

This is the voice that tells you nothing is ever good enough.

You finish a crown prep and immediately start replaying it in your mind. *Was the margin clean enough? Should I have reduced more? What if the temp falls off?*

You have a productive day and your first thought is, *sure hope we have more of these days because today's production is going entirely to bills.*

You get a compliment from a patient and you dismiss it. *They're just being nice. They don't know what good dentistry actually looks like. It's just my job.*

This voice is relentless. It does not celebrate wins. It only scans for mistakes, gaps, things you could have done better.

Research by Hewitt and Flett (1991), published in the *Journal of Personality and Social Psychology*, identified this as "self-oriented perfectionism"—setting unrealistically high standards for yourself and engaging in harsh self-criticism when you inevitably fall short. Their work showed this dimension of perfectionism is strongly associated with depression, anxiety, and burnout.

Dr. Kalli remembers being told by staff members years later, "You were really scary when you first started. We were afraid of you."

She was shocked. She was not throwing instruments. She was not yelling. But her internal standards were so high, and her frustration with herself so visible, that it created an atmosphere of tension. She was not mad at them. She was mad at herself for not being perfect. But they could not tell the difference.

2. Fear of Failure

When your worth is tied to your performance, failure is not just disappointing—it is devastating.

So you avoid situations where you might fail. You procrastinate on difficult cases. You say no to opportunities that stretch you. You stick with what you know you can do perfectly rather than risking something new.

Or you go the other direction: you overprepare to the point of exhaustion. You review the same case ten times. You research every possible complication. You rehearse the conversation you will have with the patient until you have scripted every word.

Either way, fear is driving your decisions.

Dr. Kalli describes this perfectly: "In college, I remember thinking, there's no way I can do this. And thank goodness my parents talked me off of all these ledges, because you just feel like that organic chemistry final is gonna kill you. If I don't make a good grade on this final, I'm not going to dental school. Everything felt THAT serious."

That is what fear of failure does. It turns every challenge into a life-or-death situation. It makes a bad grade feel like a character indictment. It makes a difficult case feel like proof that you are not good enough.

3. Procrastination (or Paralysis)

When the standards are impossibly high and the fear of failure is intense, your brain does something counterintuitive.

It shuts down.

You procrastinate on the very things that matter most because you know you will not be able to do them perfectly. You avoid making decisions because any decision could be the wrong one. You freeze when you should act because action carries the risk of visible failure.

Or you get stuck in analysis paralysis, endlessly gathering information, seeking more opinions, delaying treatment plans because you are waiting for absolute certainty that will never come.

Stuckness is not the same thing as laziness. It's your nervous system trying to protect you from the pain of falling short of your own impossible standards. Ferrari and colleagues (1995), in their book *Procrastination and Task Avoidance: Theory, Research, and Treatment*, demonstrated that perfectionism is one of the strongest predictors of chronic procrastination, particularly when combined with fear of negative evaluation.

And the cruel irony? The more you procrastinate, the worse you feel about yourself. The critical inner voice gets louder. The fear intensifies. And the cycle deepens.

The way out of the Triangular Trap is not to lower your standards. It is to separate your worth from your performance.

You can do excellent work without making excellence a prerequisite for self-acceptance.

You can care deeply about outcomes without making every outcome a referendum on whether you are good enough.

You can aim high without making the target impossible to hit.

But first, you have to recognize the trap you are in.

The "What If" Spiral: When Anxiety Hijacks Your Brain

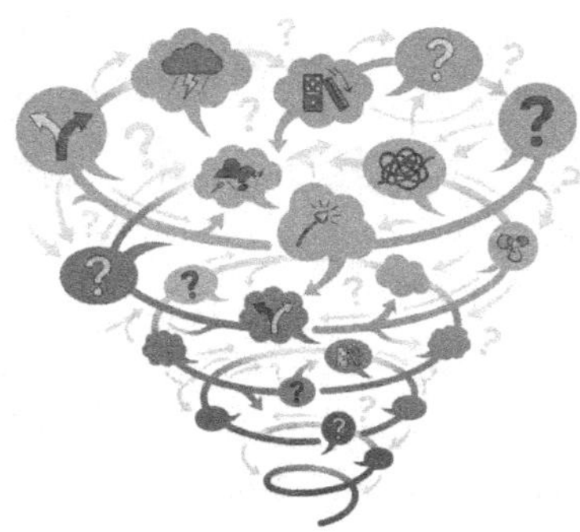

Dr. Kalli remembers lying in bed at night, unable to sleep, her mind running through the next day's schedule.

What if the crown doesn't fit?

What if the patient complains about the cost?

What if I can't get them numb?

What if they leave a bad review?

What if I fall behind schedule?

What if I miss something in the exam?

Each "what if" triggered another. And another. And another.

By the time she finally fell asleep, her nervous system was already in fight-or-flight mode. She would wake up exhausted, adrenaline already coursing through her body before she even looked at the schedule.

This is the **"What If" Spiral**, and it is one of the most common and most destructive thinking patterns among burned-out dentists.

Here is what happens neurologically:

When you think a "what if" thought about a future threat, your brain cannot tell the difference between a real danger and an imagined one. It responds the same way it would if the threat were happening right now.

Your amygdala (the fear center of your brain) activates. Your body releases adrenaline and cortisol. Your heart rate increases. Your muscles tense. Your digestion slows. Blood flow shifts away from your prefrontal cortex (the thinking, rational part of your brain) and toward your limbs (so you can fight or run).

This is the fight-or-flight response. And it is designed to save your life when you are facing an actual, immediate threat. Research by LeDoux (1996) in *The Emotional Brain* explains how the amygdala can hijack rational thinking when it perceives threat, creating a stress response before the cortex even has time to evaluate whether the threat is real.

But here is the problem.

Your brain is running this response for threats that have not happened and may never happen.

You are lying in bed at 11 p.m., and your body is reacting as if a crown that does not fit tomorrow is a saber-toothed tiger attacking you right now.

And because you are not actually running from anything, the adrenaline has nowhere to go. It just sits in your system, keeping you wired, anxious, and unable to rest.

Worse, the "what if" thinking robs you of the energy you need for the present moment. Kabat-Zinn (1990), in his foundational work *Full Catastrophe Living*, describes how catastrophic thinking about future events drains present-moment awareness and creates a chronic stress response that depletes physical and mental resources.

You spend so much mental and emotional energy worrying about what *might* go wrong tomorrow that you have nothing left for what is happening *today*. You are burned out before you even start working.

Dr. Kalli describes it this way: "When I learned this idea that your "thoughts could be false", that my own thoughts maybe aren't factual, it was like a light bulb momen 💡 for me. I was completely mind blown. Like, oh my gosh, maybe these problems are more in my mind than anywhere else.... And that was a huge pressure relief valve."

Because here is the truth most anxious, high-achieving dentists never consider:

Most of your "what if" thoughts are catastrophic predictions that never come true.

The crown fits fine.

The patient is happy with the cost.

You get them numb without issue.

They do not leave a review at all, and if they do, it is positive.

You did not miss anything in the exam.

Even if the patient was upset, you knew how to handle it and it was over quickly.

But you spent hours, maybe days, of mental energy preparing for disasters that never materialized. Stealing precious time from your life that you will never get back.

And even when something *does* go wrong, it is almost never as catastrophic as your brain predicted. You handle it. You find a solution. Life goes on.

The "what if" spiral does not protect you. It just exhausts you.

The Prove-Yourself Cycle: Why You Can't Earn Your Way Out

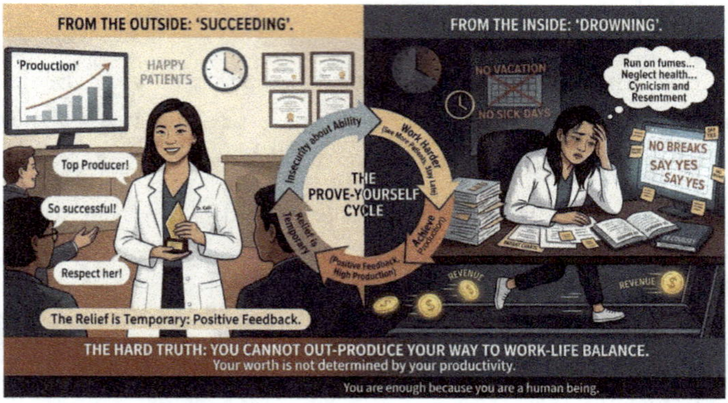
FROM THE OUTSIDE: 'SUCCEEDING'.
FROM THE INSIDE: 'DROWNING'.
'Production'
HAPPY PATIENTS
Top Producer!
So successful!
Respect her!
The Relief is Temporary: Positive Feedback.
Insecurity about Ability
Work Harder
Achieve Production
(Positive Feedback, High Production)
Relief is Temporary
THE PROVE-YOURSELF CYCLE
NO VACATION
NO SICK DAYS
Run on fumes... Neglect health... Cynicism and Resentment
NO BREAKS
SAY YES
SAY YES
REVENUE
REVENUE
THE HARD TRUTH: YOU CANNOT OUT-PRODUCE YOUR WAY TO WORK-LIFE BALANCE.
Your worth is not determined by your productivity.
You are enough because you are a human being.

One of the most insidious aspects of burnout is the **prove-yourself cycle.**

It works like this:

You feel insecure about your ability to succeed (maybe because of perfectionism, maybe because of external validation seeking, maybe because of comparison to others).

So you work harder to make it work. You see more patients. You take more CE courses. You produce more revenue. You stay later. You say yes to everything. After all, you have payroll to make.

And for a while, it goes well. You get positive feedback. Patients are happy. Your production numbers go up. Colleagues respect you.

But the relief is temporary.

Because the busy season never ends.

No matter how much you achieve, the boundaries you lack put you back in the rat race at work.. The fear that you will never be able to miss a day at the office, be sick, or spontaneously go on vacation, is palpable. This is where the cynicism and resentment really started to set in for Dr. Kalli

Before you know it you are running on fumes, neglecting your health, missing time with your family, and wondering why you feel so horribly stressed despite how well you are doing YOUR job.

Maslach and Leiter (1997), in their seminal work *The Truth About Burnout*, describe this as one of the core pathways to burnout: the mismatch between effort and reward. When you believe you must constantly prove your success through achievement (i.e. how successful your practice is), you create an exhausting cycle where the goalposts keep moving and satisfaction remains perpetually out of reach.

Dr. Kalli lived this. Her practices were thriving. She was one of the top providers. She got awards at annual meetings. From the outside, she had made it.

But inside, she felt like she was drowning. The nonstop patients, abusive schedule, and not having another provider to lighten the load was suffocating. She was held on a pedestal for her achievements in dentistry, yet no one but her family knew she was about to quit.

The "prove-yourself" cycle is not about achievement. It is about trying to earn love, acceptance, or worth through performance.

And that is a game you can never win.

Here is the hard truth: **You cannot out-produce your way to better work-life balance. You cannot out-perform your way to feeling happier.**

You have to do the internal work of recognizing that your worth is not determined by your productivity, your case acceptance rate, your reviews, your office success, or how many patients you see in a day.

You are enough because you are a human being. You cannot possibly take care of your patients well if you are not taking care of yourself well. You need breaks in your day. You need to eat lunch, drink water, and schedule your patients in a way that fuels your talent, not depletes it.

The work you do is valuable and the fact that you are reading this says more about how much you care than anything else. But, your work is not what makes *you* valuable.

And until you believe that—really believe it, not just intellectually but in your bones—you will keep pushing yourself into burnout. And burnout will limit what you are capable of achieving: freedom in your work day, increased productivity, and a career that lasts.

The False Belief: "If I Just Work Harder..."

There is a lie that high-achieving dentists tell themselves.

If I just work harder, I can get through this.

This belief is baked into dental training. You survived dental school by working harder. You built your practice by working harder. You have solved most problems in your career by putting in more effort.

So when stress increases, when the schedule gets overwhelming, when burnout starts creeping in, your instinct is to do what has always worked before.

Push harder. Work longer. See more patients. Say yes to more opportunities.

But here is what the research shows, and what Dr. Kalli learned the hard way:

Working harder when you are already burned out makes everything worse.

A landmark study by Pencavel (2014), published by the Stanford Institute for Economic Policy Research, analyzed productivity data and found that output per hour declines sharply when the work week exceeds 50 hours, and productivity drops so precipitously after 55 hours that working additional time produces negligible output. In fact, someone working 70 hours produces little more than someone working 55 hours—the extra 15 hours are essentially wasted effort that only increases fatigue and health risks.

More importantly, research by Perlow and Porter (2009) in the *Harvard Business Review* showed that professionals who set hard boundaries and "logged off" mentally from work reported higher productivity scores and better work quality than those who remained constantly available. They called this "predictable time off"—and it dramatically improved both performance and wellbeing.

Why?

Because your brain needs rest to function well. Your nervous system needs recovery time. Your body needs sleep, nutrition, and movement that are not squeezed into the margins of an impossible schedule.

When you are already past The Hump on the Human Function Curve, more effort produces worse results.

Dr. Kalli was working four full days a week, seeing 140 new patients a month, skipping bathroom breaks, barely eating lunch. She was producing excellent work. But she was also losing her hair. Her blood pressure was in crisis territory. She was irritable at home. She could not sleep. She was one bad day away from quitting entirely.

And when her husband, Dr. Kyle, finally forced her to cut a day, when she blocked off Tuesdays and committed to *not being in the building*, something counterintuitive happened.

Her quality of life improved dramatically. And her practice did not fall apart.

In fact, once she hired more help and created better systems, the practice thrived. Because she was no longer the bottleneck. She was no longer trying to do everything herself while running on adrenaline and willpower.

Here is the principle you need to internalize:

Boundaries increase productivity. Rest improves performance. Recovery is not a luxury. It's a requirement for sustainable excellence.

Working harder is not the answer. Working smarter, with systems that protect your capacity, is.

People-Pleasing and the Word You Can't Say

Dr. Kalli describes herself in the height of burnout as someone who "just wanted to be the provider."

She wanted to help people. She wanted to deliver excellent care. She wanted every patient to have a great experience.

This is beautiful. This is why she became a dentist.

But it also meant she could not say no.

When a patient messaged her on Facebook at 9 p.m. about Zoom whitening, she answered. Because saying "that can wait until business hours" felt rude.

When staff asked her to stay late to fit in an emergency, she said yes. Because saying "we need to establish protocols for emergencies so this doesn't happen every day" felt selfish.

When her schedule was triple-booked with no breaks, she pushed through. Because saying "this is not sustainable and we need to redesign how we schedule" felt like letting people down.

She was saying yes to everyone else and no to herself. No to her family. Over and over and over.

And people-pleasing feels noble when you are doing it. It feels like compassion. Like service. Like being a good doctor.

But it is not sustainable.

Because eventually, you run out. You become what Dr. Kalli calls "a stump"—like the tree in Shel Silverstein's classic children's book *The Giving Tree* (1964) that gave and gave and gave until there was nothing left.

Here is the hard truth about people-pleasing:

It is not actually about caring for others. It is about avoiding the discomfort of disappointing them.

When you cannot say no, it is not because you are so compassionate. It is because you are afraid of what will happen if you set a boundary. Afraid they will be upset. Afraid they will leave a bad review. Afraid they will think you do not care. Afraid they will leave your practice.

And sometimes those fears are valid. Sometimes patients *will* be upset. Sometimes they *will* leave.

But here is what Dr. Kalli learned: **You cannot build a sustainable practice by sacrificing yourself to keep everyone happy.**

The patients who need you to be available 24/7 are not your ideal patients. The staff members who expect you to tolerate poor performance because you are afraid to fire them are not helping you build something great. The insurance companies that demand you work for reimbursement rates that do not cover your costs do not have your best interests at heart.

Saying no is not selfish. It is self-preservation. It is leadership. It is the only way to create space for the people and work that truly matter. It's the only way to create space for you.

Dr. Kalli eventually blocked Tuesdays. She stopped answering messages after hours. She got out of network with insurance. She set expectations with her team about what was acceptable and what was not.

And some patients left. Some staff members were upset. Some people thought she was being difficult.

But the patients who stayed were the ones she actually wanted to serve. The staff who adapted became her strongest team members. And she built a practice she did not want to escape from. In fact, it ALL worked out.

Healthy selflessness is not about doing everything for everyone. It is about doing your best for the people you are meant to serve without sacrificing yourself in the process.

This concept of healthy boundaries in helping professions has been explored extensively by Figley (1995) in his work on compassion fatigue. In *Compassion Fatigue: Coping with Secondary Traumatic Stress Disorder in Those Who Treat the Traumatized*, he describes how caregivers who cannot set boundaries eventually experience emotional depletion that prevents them from providing quality care—essentially, unlimited giving ultimately harms both the giver and those they serve.

Real Talk: Control Issues and the Delegation Barrier

If you are reading this and thinking, *Okay, but I can't just hand things off to other people because they won't do it right,* then we need to talk about control.

Dentists are trained to be in control. You control the procedure. You control the outcome. You control every detail because precision matters and mistakes have consequences.

This is appropriate in the operatory.

It becomes a problem when you extend it to everything else.

Dr. Kalli describes watching some of the dentists she mentors struggle with delegation: "Why are you the one picking up the phone to call the lab to figure out where that case is? That makes no sense. You are hiring people to work for you. You have a great assistant. You have a treatment coordinator team. When they ask you a question like, 'Hey, where's this case?' put it right back to them. 'We need a system for tracking cases. Call the lab for me. Keep me updated.'"

But dentists resist this. Because what if the assistant does not call the right person? What if they do not ask the right questions? What if the lab gives them incorrect information and the assistant does not catch it? Or maybe you assume you're imposing on your employee who is "busy with other things".

So instead of delegating, you do it yourself. You add it to your mental load. You stay late making phone calls that someone else should be making. You micromanage every detail because you are convinced that if you do not control it, it will fall apart.

And maybe in the beginning, when you had five patients a week, you could do everything yourself.

But now you have 140 new patients a month. You have four hygienists. You have multiple operatories running simultaneously. You have staff asking you questions every five minutes.

And you are still trying to control everything.

That is not excellence. That is a recipe for burnout.

Here is what control issues actually are: **fear dressed up as responsibility.**

You are afraid that if you let go, something will go wrong. You are afraid that if someone else does it, they will make a mistake and it will reflect poorly on you. You are afraid that if you are not indispensable, you will lose value.

Research on workplace autonomy supports this. Karasek and Theorell (1990) in *Healthy Work: Stress, Productivity, and the Reconstruction of Working Life* identified that high demands combined with low control creates the most toxic work environment for burnout. Ironically, dentists often create their own low-control environment by refusing to delegate—they increase their demands while simultaneously limiting their actual control over outcomes.

But the truth is this: **You cannot scale by doing everything yourself. You cannot build a sustainable practice by being the bottleneck.**

Dr. Kalli learned this the hard way. She had to train her team to handle things without her. She had to tolerate the discomfort of things not being done exactly the way she would do them. She had to accept that delegating meant occasional mistakes, and that those mistakes were not catastrophic.

And once she did, she got her life back.

Because delegation is not about lowering standards. It is about empowering other people to meet high standards so you do not have to carry everything alone.

The Gift You Didn't Ask For

Here is the paradox of the Type A trap.

The traits that make you vulnerable to burnout—perfectionism, high responsibility, relentless work ethic, care for others—are also the traits that make you an excellent dentist.

You cannot just "turn off" your conscientiousness. You cannot stop caring about outcomes. You cannot lower your standards and still feel like you are doing good work.

So the solution is not to change who you are. The solution is to build systems that protect you from the extremes of who you are. Systems that force you to delegate even when it is uncomfortable. Boundaries that prevent you from over-giving. Self-awareness that helps you notice when perfectionism has crossed into self-sabotage. Mental tools that interrupt the "what if" spiral before it hijacks your nervous system.

You do not need to become a different person. You need to learn how to be who you are—conscientious, driven, caring—in a way that does not destroy you.

And that is exactly what the rest of this book is about.

But first, we need to talk about the unique pressures of dentistry itself. Because it is not just what you bring to the chair that creates burnout. It is also what dentistry demands from you—physically, mentally, emotionally, and financially—that makes this profession uniquely difficult.

That is what we turn to next.

Reflection Questions:

1. Which part of the Triangular Trap do you recognize most in yourself: the critical inner voice, fear of failure, or procrastination/paralysis?
2. What "what if" thoughts do you replay most often? How much of your mental energy goes to scenarios that never happen?
3. What would it feel like to believe that your success is not determined by your productivity?

4. Where are you saying yes when you need to say no? What are you afraid will happen if you set that boundary?

References for Chapter 2:

Ferrari, J. R., Johnson, J. L., & McCown, W. G. (1995). *Procrastination and task avoidance: Theory, research, and treatment.* Springer.

Figley, C. R. (Ed.). (1995). *Compassion fatigue: Coping with secondary traumatic stress disorder in those who treat the traumatized.* Brunner/Mazel.

Hewitt, P. L., & Flett, G. L. (1991). Perfectionism in the self and social contexts: Conceptualization, assessment, and association with psychopathology. *Journal of Personality and Social Psychology, 60*(3), 456-470.

Hill, A. P., & Curran, T. (2016). Multidimensional perfectionism and burnout: A meta-analysis. *Personality and Social Psychology Review, 20*(3), 269-288.

Kabat-Zinn, J. (1990). *Full catastrophe living: Using the wisdom of your body and mind to face stress, pain, and illness.* Delacorte Press.

Karasek, R., & Theorell, T. (1990). *Healthy work: Stress, productivity, and the reconstruction of working life.* Basic Books.

LeDoux, J. (1996). *The emotional brain: The mysterious underpinnings of emotional life.* Simon & Schuster.

Maslach, C., & Leiter, M. P. (1997). *The truth about burnout: How organizations cause personal stress and what to do about it.* Jossey-Bass.

Pencavel, J. (2014). *The productivity of working hours.* Stanford Institute for Economic Policy Research Discussion Paper No. 14-004.

Perlow, L. A., & Porter, J. L. (2009). Making time off predictable—and required. *Harvard Business Review, 87*(10), 102-109.

Silverstein, S. (1964). *The giving tree.* Harper & Row.

Swider, B. W., & Zimmerman, R. D. (2010). Born to burnout: A meta-analytic path model of personality, job burnout, and work outcomes. *Journal of Vocational Behavior, 76*(3), 487-506.

CHAPTER 3

Blue-Collar Work In A White Coat

Dr. Kalli Hale's father has a phrase he uses to describe dentistry.

"Dentistry is blue-collar work masked in a white coat."

He means this literally. You are on your feet all day. Your back hurts. Your neck is stiff. Your hands cramp. You are bent over someone's mouth for hours, holding instruments, applying pressure, maintaining precision in awkward positions that would make an ergonomics specialist cringe.

But you are also wearing a white coat. Making what people assume is "white coat money." Expected to project professionalism, authority, expertise. Expected to own a nice car, live in a nice house, take nice vacations.

The dissonance between these two realities—physical labor that grinds your body down combined with cognitive demands that drain your brain and financial expectations that keep you on a treadmill—is part of what makes dental burnout so uniquely brutal.

Most people do not understand what you actually do all day. Honestly, only a dentist could. They see the degree. They see the title. They assume you have it figured out. They have no idea.

I like to pretend that if they DID understand, they would treat all of us with more grace.

The Unique Stressors of Dental Practice

Every profession has stress. But dentistry combines stressors in a way that few other careers do.

You work in one of the most vulnerable spaces on the human body. The mouth is intimate. It's personal. It's associated with pain and fear and childhood trauma. Most of your patients do not want to be there. They are anxious before you even start. And you have to manage their fear while simultaneously performing precise, irreversible procedures.

You make hundreds of micro-decisions every single day. Is this decay? Do I watch it or treat it? What material should I use? Did I reduce enough? Which anesthetic? What if they react poorly? Every choice has consequences—clinical, financial, legal. And you make them constantly, all day, with limited time to deliberate.

You are responsible for outcomes you do not fully control. You can do everything right—perfect prep, perfect restoration, perfect follow-up—and the patient still might not be happy. The crown might not feel right to them. The occlusion might be off by a fraction of a millimeter that only they can perceive. Or they might not follow your post-op instructions and blame you when something goes wrong.

You manage physical pain, emotional fear, and financial expectations simultaneously. You are trying to get someone numb while they are gripping the armrests and sweating. You are explaining treatment while they are worried about cost. You are working in a two-inch space with limited visibility while your patient is convinced you are going to hurt them. This is not normal work. This is emotional labor layered on top of physical and cognitive labor.

You are only as good as your last patient interaction. One bad experience, one miscommunication, one moment where you seemed rushed or dismissive, and you could end up with a one-star review that lives on Google forever. Your reputation is constantly on the line.

Dr. Kalli describes the relentless nature of it this way: "When you're a dentist, you are constantly hit with questions and problems—they are not all crisis-level, but every single thing is something you have to fix and address for the *entire* time you are in the building."

There is no downtime. No transition between tasks. You finish one procedure, walk into the next operatory, and immediately have to shift gears—new patient, new problem, new decisions, new emotional regulation required.

And this happens for eight hours straight. Four days a week. Fifty weeks a year.

For decades.

Decision Fatigue: The Invisible Drain

Decision fatigue is one of the most underestimated contributors to dental burnout.

Every decision you make, no matter how small, depletes a finite mental resource. By the end of the day, your ability to make good decisions deteriorates. You become more impulsive, more avoidant, more likely to stick with the default option even when it is not the best choice.

And dentistry is nothing but decisions.

Before you even see your first patient, you are making decisions. What teeth are we treating today? Did I review the medical history yet? Will my assistant remember to take blood pressure?

Then the patient sits down.

Do I see recurrent decay under this filling? How deep is it? Did I warn this patient they might need endo? What material should I use? Infiltration or block? Articaine or lidocaine? How much reduction? Is this enough? Too much? This is going to take longer than I blocked. Can I handle it? What's my contingency plan? If I run behind, the next patient waiting is going to be upset.

And that is just one tooth. One patient. One appointment.

Multiply that by ten patients. Twenty patients. Thirty patients.

By the time you get to your last patient of the day, your decision-making capacity is gone. You are running on autopilot. Your brain is fried.

And then you go home and your spouse asks, "What do you want for dinner?" and you feel a wave of irritation because you do not have one more decision left in you.

Dr. Kalli remembers days when she would come home and just need to sit in silence. Not because she did not love her family. But because her brain had been making high-stakes decisions for eight hours and she had nothing left to give.

Decision fatigue does not just make you tired. It makes you worse at your job. It increases the likelihood of errors. It reduces your ability to communicate effectively with patients. It makes you more likely to say yes when you should say no, or avoid a difficult conversation that needs to happen.

And because you are conscientious and care about quality, you compensate by working even harder. Reviewing cases at night. Second-guessing yourself. Replaying decisions to make sure you did not miss anything. Wondering if the patient "liked" you or not.

Which only makes the fatigue worse.

Physical Labor Meets Cognitive Precision

Dentistry is one of the few professions that demands sustained physical exertion and extreme cognitive precision at the same time.

You are not just standing. You are bent over at an awkward angle. Holding instruments that require fine motor control. Applying pressure. Maintaining stability. For minutes at a time. Then hours at a time.

Your neck is flexed forward. Your shoulders are rounded. Your lower back is compressed. Your hands are locked in awkward positions.

And while your body is under this physical strain, your brain is performing microsurgery.

You are working in a space the size of a walnut, trying to remove decay without hitting the pulp, trying to shape a prep without overreducing, trying to place a margin subgingivally while your patient is gagging or bleeding or moving their tongue. Or you're having a serious conversation with someone about how you have to pull all of their teeth. Talk about emotional!

This is not a task you can do half-focused. You cannot let your mind wander. One wrong move and you have a pulp exposure, a fractured tooth, a perforated canal.

So you are physically exhausted and mentally hyper-vigilant. At the same time. All day.

And unlike surgery, where you scrub out after a case and get a break, you finish one procedure and immediately walk into the next operatory where another patient is waiting.

Dr. Kalli remembers days when she did not take a bathroom break. Did not drink water. Did not sit down. Just moved from chair to chair, patient to patient, case to case, until the last one was done.

She was not being heroic. She was surviving. Because if she stopped, she would fall behind. And if she fell behind, patients would be waiting. And if patients were waiting, they would be unhappy. And if they were unhappy, they might leave a bad review.

So she kept going.

Until her body forced her to stop.

The 186/120 blood pressure reading was not random. It was her body screaming, "You cannot keep doing this."

Managing Pain, Fear, and Expectations Simultaneously

A patient sits down. They are sighing, visibly anxious. Their jaw is tense. They are breathing shallowly. Before you even say hello, they tell you, "I hate the dentist. I had a bad experience as a kid. No one can ever get me numb."

Now you have to do several things at once:

1. Calm them down so they can relax enough for you to work.
2. Build trust so they will actually follow your treatment recommendations.
3. Perform a clinical procedure with precision and care.
4. Manage the clock because you have other patients waiting.
5. Anticipate their financial concerns and prepare for the cost conversation.

And you have to do all of this while projecting confidence, competence, and calm—even if you are stressed, behind schedule, or dealing with your own problems.

This is why Dr. Kalli talks about the importance of body language and tone. "I'm really big on body language. I really feel like if you start paying attention to what your body language is to the patient, you will help them to relax and vice versa. If they're really stressed or they're really tense, I might be sitting a little straight in the beginning too, but I'm going to start talking a bit slower. I'm going to be taking some deep breaths and we're going to bring the tension down in the room."

This requires immense self-regulation. You cannot be reactive. You cannot show frustration. You cannot let your own stress leak into the interaction. You actually have to create space between what's happening and how you navigate the conversation. Major self awareness.

You have to be the calm one. The reassuring one. The one who has it together. Even when you do not.

And then, on top of managing the patient's fear and pain, you also have to manage their expectations.

They want it done fast. They want it to be cheap. They want it to look perfect. They want zero discomfort. And they want you to guarantee the outcome.

Which is impossible. But you still have to navigate that conversation with empathy and professionalism. Oh, and make money.

Every. Single. Day.

The Insurance Trap and Production Pressure

Speaking of money…

If you are in-network with dental insurance, you are dealing with one of the most frustrating aspects of modern dentistry: reimbursement rates that barely cover your costs.

Dr. Kalli remembers the years she spent in-network. "Some plans only pay $37 for a cleaning and your hygienist is $50 an hour? You need to identify which insurance company you cannot afford to take anymore, because you literally can't, and drop it."

Let that sink in.

Insurance pays you $37. Your hygienist costs you $50 per hour. You are losing money on every cleaning.

But if you drop the insurance, patients might leave. And if patients leave, your schedule has holes. And if your schedule has holes, you are not producing. And if you are not producing, you cannot make payroll.

So you stay in-network. You see more patients to make up the difference. You pack your schedule tighter and tighter, trying to make the math work.

And it grinds you down.

Even if you are out-of-network, there is still production pressure. Because you have overhead. Staff salaries, lab fees, rent, equipment, supplies, loan payments. And all of that comes out before you take home a single dollar.

So you are constantly aware of the numbers. How much did I produce today? How much did we collect? Are we on track for the month? Can I make payroll? Can I afford to hire help?

The business side of dentistry is relentless. And most dentists were never trained for it.

Dr. Kalli puts it bluntly: "You have absolutely no business training in dental school. This is a big problem. You have absolutely no financial advice, financial discussions for the massive hundreds of thousands of dollars of student loans you have. Then you're being sold every shiny toy for your office. You're in tons of debt. And you feel like you cannot get out."

So you are trying to be a great clinician, a great leader, a great business owner, and a great human being all while drowning in debt and trying to figure out how to make the numbers work.

It is suffocating.

Practice Ownership vs. Associateship: Different Burnout, Same Result

Dr. Kalli works with both practice owners and associates. And she has seen burnout destroy both.

Practice owners burn out from the weight of responsibility. Everything falls on you. Payroll, HR, marketing, operations, staff conflicts, patient complaints, equipment failures, regulatory compliance, and insurance negotiations.

You are the dentist, the CEO, the HR manager, the marketing director, and the janitor when something breaks after hours.

You cannot just clock out and go home. The practice is always with you. In your mind. In your stress. In your bank account.

And if you are the kind of person who cannot delegate (which most dentists are), you try to do everything yourself. Which means you are working clinically all day and then handling business tasks at night and on weekends.

Associates burn out from lack of control. You do not own the practice, so you do not get to make the rules. Someone else sets your schedule. Someone else decides what insurance you take. Someone else hires your assistant.

And if you work for a corporate entity or a high-volume practice, the pressure to produce is relentless. You are measured by numbers. Judged by productivity. Expected to meet quotas that may not align with the kind of care you want to provide.

Dr. Kalli describes the associates she has hired over the years: "The number one complaint we get from associates wanting to leave wherever they are is they either do not have enough resources—they can't make decisions about letting an assistant go that's not doing well—or they really want to leave at 3pm and go pick up their kids. They've been out for 10 years, they've done their hustle and grind, but they're done staying until the last patient of the day."

So whether you own the practice or work for someone else, the burnout is real. Owners burn out from too much responsibility. Associates burn out from too little autonomy.

Same result. Same exhaustion. Same desire to just walk away.

The Hustle You Didn't Sign Up For: From Dental School to Financial Quicksand

Let's talk about the pipeline that leads to burnout.

It starts in high school. You are a high achiever. You get straight A's because anything less feels like failure. You sacrifice social life, sleep, fun—because you have a goal. You want to be a dentist.

Then college. Pre-dental track. Every exam matters. Every grade could determine whether you get into dental school. Organic chemistry. Physics. Biology. You are competing against other high achievers, and the stakes feel life-or-death.

You get in. Dental school. You made it.

Except now the pressure intensifies. You are drowning in material. Barely sleeping. Taking exams that determine whether you pass or fail, whether you stay or get cut. You watch classmates—smart, capable people—leave because they could not handle it.

Dr. Kalli's class started with 88 students. Six did not finish.

And the entire time, you are accumulating debt. Student loans that grow every semester. Loans you try not to think about because if you do, the number is so big it feels insurmountable.

Then you graduate. You think the hard part is over.

It is not.

Because now you are $300,000 in debt (or more). You need to find a job. You need to start paying back loans. You are competing for positions. You are trying to build a patient base from scratch. You are learning how to actually practice dentistry—because dental school taught you techniques, not real-world problem-solving.

And you are doing this with zero business training. Zero financial literacy. Zero understanding of how to manage staff, market a practice, negotiate with insurance companies, or design systems that protect your wellbeing.

So you do what you have always done. You work hard. You say yes to everything. You grind.

And the grind works. For a while. You build a patient base. You start producing. The numbers go up.

But so does the stress. The schedule gets packed. The responsibilities pile up. The debt is still there. The pressure to keep producing is constant.

And before you know it, you are in your mid-thirties, successful on paper, burned out in reality, wondering how you ended up here. Sadly, perhaps because of this, the suicide rate in dentistry is very high. Being a dentist literally doubles the statistical likelihood that suicide will be the cause of death compared to your neighbors (according to research by Dr. Suzanne Tomasi and colleagues, published in the *Journal of the American Dental Association*).

That's why we wanted this book to be not just about ways to save the profession but to save your life.

We refuse to let these statistics be the final word on your career. To change the numbers, we have to change the way we work—starting right now.

In the next section, we move from diagnosis to treatment. We stop talking about what is wrong and start talking about what to do about it. Because you cannot think your way out of burnout. You have to act your way out. And the first step is stabilization—stopping the acute bleeding before you can rebuild.

That is where we go next.

Reflection Questions:

1. Which aspect of the "blue-collar work in a white coat" dynamic do you feel most acutely: the physical toll, the decision fatigue, the emotional labor, or the financial pressure?
2. When you feel overwhelmed, what is your default response? Do you push harder, or do you pause and reassess the system?
3. If you could redesign one aspect of your workday to reduce the grind, what would it be?
4. What would it take for you to believe that working smarter (not harder) is the answer?

PART II
Stabilization & Treatment

CHAPTER 4

Stop The Bleeding: Acute Burnout Stabilization

There is a moment in every crisis when you realize you cannot keep going the way you have been.

For Dr. Kalli Hale, that moment came on an ordinary Thursday afternoon. The dizziness, then the blood pressure spike.

That moment—that undeniable, physiological evidence that she was in crisis—was what finally broke through the denial.

What was your "186 over 120" moment? You know the one. It's the moment where the "fine" you've been telling yourself finally rings hollow. Maybe it wasn't a blood pressure cuff. Maybe it was the morning you sat in your car in the parking lot, gripping the steering wheel, unable to force your legs to move toward the front door. Maybe it was the sudden, hot flash of uncharacteristic rage at your employee's simple question, or the way your hands started shaking during a routine crown prep.

It's that split second where you realize you can no longer pretend that this level of stress is just "the cost of doing business."

If you are reading this because you are in that place—if your body is sending signals you've been ignoring, or if you are one bad day away from walking out—then this chapter is your emergency triage. We are not here to fix your entire life today. We are here to stop the bleeding.

Because you cannot rebuild while you are still actively breaking down.

Emergency Triage: When You're in Crisis

If you are in acute burnout—if you are physically, mentally, or emotionally at your breaking point—you need to understand something critical.

This is not the time for a five-year plan. This is the time for a tourniquet.

You do not need to redesign your entire practice right now. You do not need to implement complex systems. You do not need to read ten books and take three courses.

You need to stabilize. Immediately.

Here is how to know if you are in crisis:

Physical symptoms that cannot be ignored:

- Chest pain, heart palpitations, or irregular heartbeat
- Severely elevated blood pressure (like Dr. Kalli's 186/120)
- Chronic insomnia that persists despite exhaustion
- Panic attacks or sudden, overwhelming anxiety, dizziness
- Physical pain that has no clear medical cause (chronic headaches, digestive issues, unexplained muscle tension)
- Extreme fatigue that does not improve with rest

Mental and emotional symptoms:

- You have serious, recurrent thoughts about quitting dentistry entirely
- You fantasize about your practice failing so you have an "excuse" to leave
- You feel numb or disconnected from patients, staff, and your own life
- You cannot remember the last time you felt joy or satisfaction from your work
- You are irritable or reactive in ways that are out of character for you
- You feel hopeless about your situation ever improving
- You fantasize about something bad happening so you don't have to go into the office

Behavioral red flags:

- You are making uncharacteristic mistakes in clinical work
- You are avoiding patient interactions or difficult conversations
- You are self-medicating with alcohol, food, or other substances to cope
- You have withdrawn from relationships and activities you used to enjoy
- You are working constantly but accomplishing less

If you checked multiple items on that list, you are not "just stressed." You are in burnout crisis.

And the first step is acknowledging that this is an emergency.

Not tomorrow. Not next month when things calm down. Now.

Recognizing the Early Warning Signs (Before the Crisis Hits)

Dr. Kalli's blood pressure crisis did not come out of nowhere. Her body had been sending signals for months. She just was not listening.

Most dentists are exceptionally good at ignoring their bodies. You have trained yourself to override physical signals. You hold your bladder for hours. You skip meals. You work through pain. You push through fatigue.

This ability to override discomfort is part of what made you successful in dental school. But it is also what makes you vulnerable to burnout. Because your body is constantly giving you feedback. You are just not listening.

Here are the early warning signs—the symptoms that show up *before* you hit crisis numbers on a blood pressure cuff:

The adrenaline spike when you look at your schedule. You open your practice management software to see what the day looks like, and immediately your heart starts racing. Your shoulders tense. Your jaw clenches.

This is not normal. This is a stress response. Your brain is perceiving the schedule as a threat.

The knot in your stomach on Sunday night. You cannot enjoy your day off because you are already dreading Monday. You feel nauseous, anxious, irritable.

This is not "just part of having a job." This is chronic anticipatory stress.

The inability to relax even when you have time. You finally have a day off, but you cannot settle. You are restless. Your mind is racing. You feel guilty for not being productive.

This is nervous system dysregulation. Your body has forgotten how to shift into rest mode.

The need for alcohol, food, or other substances to "take the edge off." You find yourself needing a drink every night. Or eating to soothe stress. Or relying on caffeine to function and sleep aids to rest.

This is not self-care. This is self-medication. And it is a sign that your nervous system needs real recovery, not numbing.

The emotional volatility. You snap at your spouse over nothing. You cry in the car. You feel rage at minor inconveniences. Or you feel nothing at all, just numb.

This is emotional dysregulation caused by chronic stress. When your nervous system is maxed out, you lose the ability to modulate your responses.

The physical pain you attribute to "just getting older." Your neck hurts. Your back hurts. Your hands ache. You tell yourself it is just the nature of the job.

But pain is a signal. And chronic pain is a sign that your body is under sustained stress.

The increasing difficulty concentrating during procedures. You catch yourself zoning out mid-prep. You have to recheck your work multiple times because you are not confident you did it right. You forget what you were about to say to the patient.

This is cognitive fatigue. Your brain is running on fumes.

The sensation of going through the motions. You are doing your job competently, but you feel like you are watching yourself from outside your body. There is no joy. No engagement. Just mechanical movement through the day.

This is dissociation, one of the early signs of depersonalization in burnout.

Start paying attention to these signals. Not to judge yourself. Not to add one more thing to your list. But to gather data.

Your body is trying to tell you something. And the sooner you listen, the less dramatic the intervention needs to be.

The goal is to catch burnout at the "adrenaline spike when you check the schedule" phase, not at the "186/120 in the middle of a conversation" phase.

What Your Body Is Actually Telling You

When you experience these symptoms, here is what is happening physiologically:

Elevated heart rate and muscle tension: Your sympathetic nervous system (fight-or-flight) is stuck in the "on" position. Your body thinks you are in constant danger. It is flooding you with stress hormones—cortisol, adrenaline—that are designed for short-term survival, not long-term functioning.

Insomnia and disrupted sleep: Your body cannot rest because your nervous system is hypervigilant. Even when you are physically exhausted, your brain stays activated, scanning for threats, replaying scenarios, anticipating problems.

Digestive issues: When you are in chronic stress, your body shuts down non-essential systems like digestion to conserve energy for survival. This is why so many burned-out dentists have stomach problems, nausea, or appetite changes.

Chronic pain: Your body is literally bracing for impact all day, every day. Your muscles never fully relax. Over time, this creates chronic pain in your neck, shoulders, back, and jaw.

These are not minor inconveniences. These are your body's desperate attempts to get you to stop before you cause irreversible damage.

If your body is sending you warning signals, listen.

Do not wait until you hit crisis numbers. Intervene now, while the symptoms are still manageable.

Immediate Interventions That Work in the Operatory

Here are some strategies you can use to reset, ground yourself, release the pressure, and find that emergency exit if you need it.

The 15-Second Reset Between Patients

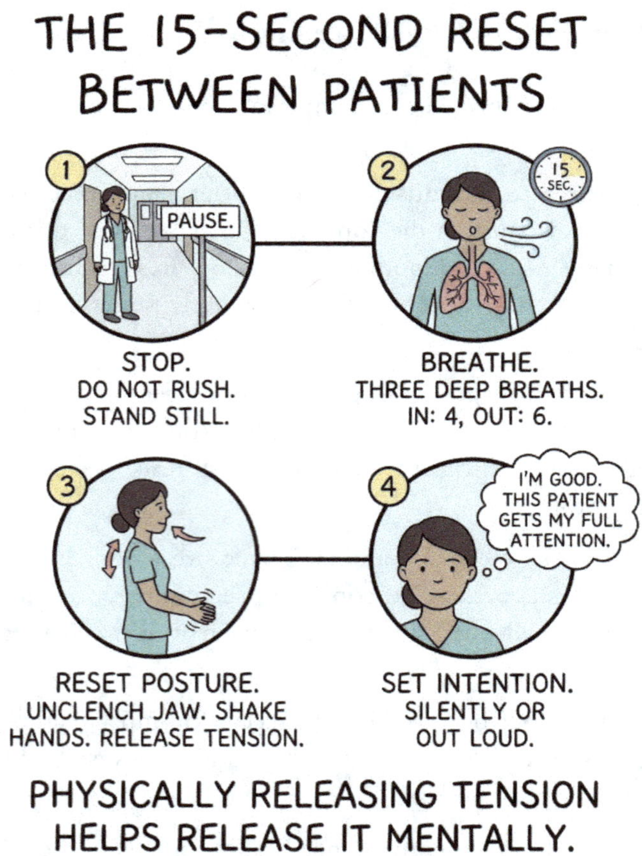

This is the single most powerful tool Dr. Kalli learned from working through *The Burnout Solution.*

Between patients—after you finish one appointment and before you walk into the next operatory—you take 15 seconds. That is it. Fifteen seconds.

Here is what you do:

Step 1: Pause. Do not immediately rush to the next room. Stop in the hallway. Stand still.

Step 2: Breathe. Three deep breaths. In through your nose for a count of four. Out through your mouth for a count of six.

This is not woo-woo. This is physiology. Slow, deep breathing activates your parasympathetic nervous system (rest-and-digest), which counteracts the stress response.

Step 3: Reset your posture. Roll your shoulders back. Unclench your jaw. Shake out your hands.

You are carrying tension in your body. Releasing it physically helps release it mentally.

Step 4: Set an intention. Say to yourself (silently or out loud): "I'm good. This patient gets my full attention."

You are not bringing the stress from the last patient into this room. You are starting fresh.

This takes fifteen seconds. And it creates a boundary between one patient and the next. A moment where you are not performing, not deciding, not fixing—just breathing.

Do this between every patient. Every single one.

It will feel impossible at first. Your brain will tell you that you do not have time, that you are already running behind, that you need to keep moving.

Do it anyway.

Because the alternative is what Dr. Kalli was doing—carrying the stress from patient one into patient two, then into patient three, compounding it all day until she was completely maxed out by the afternoon.

Fifteen seconds of reset prevents hours of recovery later.

Mantras That Ground You

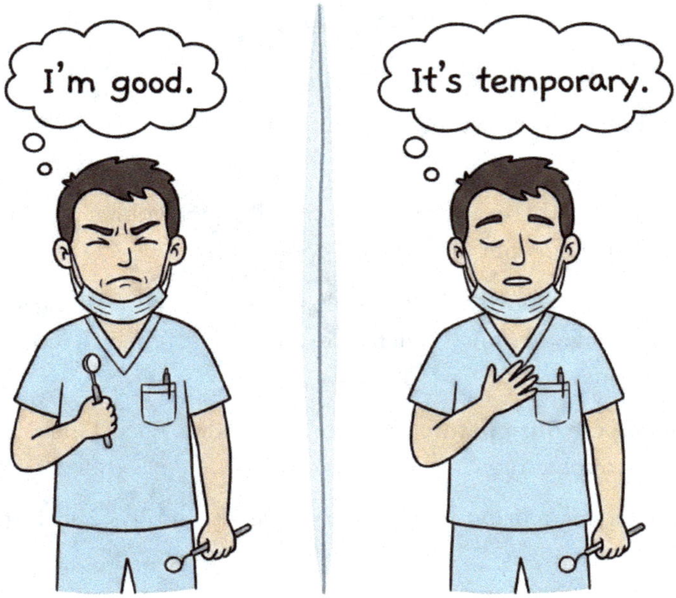

When your nervous system is in fight-or-flight, your brain is scanning for danger. It is catastrophizing. It is spiraling.

You need a way to interrupt that pattern in real time.

Dr. Kalli learned two simple phrases that became her lifeline:

"I'm good."

When something stressful happens—a patient complains, a case does not go perfectly, you are running behind—your brain wants to spiral. *Oh no, this is a disaster. They're going to leave a bad review. I'm sick of being a dentist. Everything is falling apart.*

Stop. Take a breath. Say (out loud or silently): **"I'm good."**

Not "everything is perfect." Not "this doesn't matter."

Just: "I'm good."

You are capable. You can handle this. You have handled worse. You are good.

This is not positive thinking. This is grounding. You are pulling yourself back to the present moment and reminding yourself that you are okay right now.

"It's temporary."

When you are in the thick of a hard day, it feels like it will never end. The stress feels permanent. The overwhelm feels infinite.

But it is not.

This patient will leave. This appointment will end. This day will be over. This busy season will pass. And as *The Burnout Solution* book suggests: *Never let anything affect you longer than the time it took to happen.*

This phrase does two things. First, it reminds you that feelings are not facts. The intensity you are experiencing right now will not last forever.

Second, it gives you permission to just get through it. You do not have to fix everything today. You just have to survive today.

And you can survive anything if you know it is temporary.

Dr. Kalli used these mantras constantly in the height of her burnout. When a patient messaged her on Facebook at 9 p.m., she would think, *I'm good. I can wait to respond and handle this tomorrow.*

When her schedule was triple-booked, she would think, *I'm good. This is temporary. I will redesign this next week.*

The mantras did not fix the problems. But they kept her from spiraling while she figured out the solutions.

The Mid-Day Pressure Release

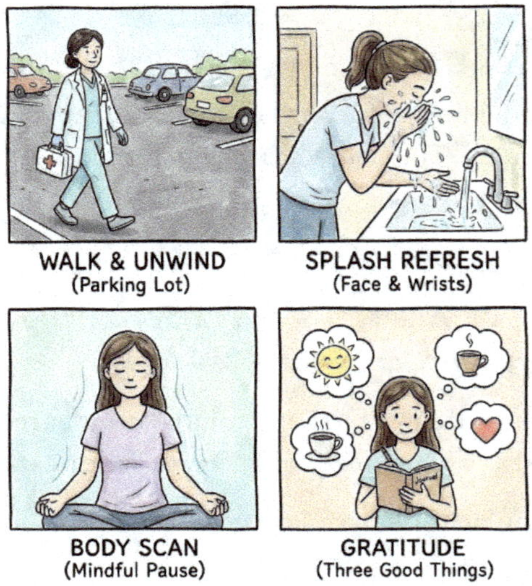

Your nervous system cannot sustain fight-or-flight for eight straight hours. It needs periodic releases.

Here are quick interventions you can use during the day when you feel yourself maxing out:

The 60-second walkabout. Step outside. Even if it is just to the parking lot. Feel the air on your face. Look at the sky. Give your brain a different visual input than operatory walls.

The cold water reset. Splash cold water on your face and wrists. The temperature change signals your nervous system to shift states. It is a physiological interrupt.

The body scan release. Close your eyes for 30 seconds. Scan your body from head to toe. Where are you holding tension? Consciously release it. Drop your shoulders. Soften your jaw. Uncurl your toes.

The gratitude redirect. Name three things that went well today. Not "everything is great." Just three specific moments. This interrupts the negativity bias that makes you focus only on what is going wrong.

These take less than a minute each. But they create micro-moments of recovery that prevent complete depletion.

The Emergency Exit Strategy

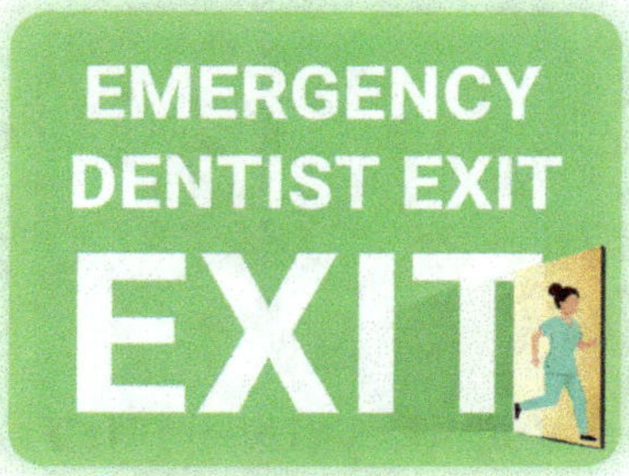

Here is something no one tells you.

You are allowed to leave.

If you are in the middle of a workday and you are having a panic attack, if you are so overwhelmed you cannot function, if you recognize the warning signs of a crisis coming on—you are allowed to stop.

You do not have to finish the day. You do not have to see every patient. You do not have to keep pushing through.

You are allowed to say, "I need to stop."

Dr. Kalli remembers the day she walked out the back door, the emergency exit, because she could not face her schedule. She looked at it—double-booked, no lunch, multiple difficult cases—and she physically could not walk into those operatories.

So she left. She went out the back door. She stood in the grass. She cried.

And Dr. Kyle came and found her. And he looked at her schedule. And he was furious—not at her, but at the system that had allowed her to be scheduled that way.

And he said, "You're not doing this. We're fixing this right now."

They had an emergency meeting with the staff. They redesigned the scheduling protocols. They blocked her schedule going forward.

But the key moment was Dr. Kalli giving herself permission to stop.

You do not have to wait for a crisis to give yourself that permission.

If you are at your breaking point, stop. Call your team together. Explain that you need help. Reschedule patients if necessary. Take a day off. Take a week off.

Your health is more important than one day's production.

And if your practice cannot survive you taking care of yourself, then the practice is broken and needs to be fixed.

Creating Your First Boundary (Even If It Terrifies You)

The first boundary is always the hardest.

Because you have spent your entire career saying yes. Yes to patients. Yes to staff. Yes to more hours, more cases, more responsibility.

And now you have to say no.

And it feels impossible, selfish, even unprofessional.

But here is the truth: **Boundaries are not selfish. They are survival.**

For Dr. Kalli, the first boundary was Tuesdays. Dr. Kyle told her, "You're cutting a day. Pick the day." And she resisted. *I can't. I'm booked six months out. Patients need me. The practice needs the revenue.*

But Dr. Kyle was firm. "We're making this happen. The schedule is going to be blocked. What are you going to do with the day?" And she picked Tuesday.

At first, it felt terrifying. She was convinced the practice would fall apart. That patients would leave. That she would lose income she could not afford to lose.

None of that happened. Funny how your mind can lie to you. The practice adapted. Patients rescheduled. The team figured it out. And Dr. Kalli got one day a week where she could breathe.

Here is how to create your first boundary:

1. Identify the thing that is killing you. What is the one thing that, if it changed, would give you the most relief?

Is it the schedule? The after-hours messages? The lack of lunch breaks? The constant interruptions? Pick one thing.

2. Decide what the boundary looks like. Be specific. Not "I need better work-life balance." That is too vague.

Instead:

- "I will not answer patient messages after 6 p.m."
- "I will block one day per week for non-clinical work."
- "I will take a 30-minute lunch break every day, no exceptions."
- "I will not be in the building on my day off."

Make it concrete and measurable.

3. Communicate it clearly. Tell your team. Tell your patients (or have your team tell them). Put it in writing if necessary.

Do not apologize. Do not over-explain. Just state it as a fact.

"Starting next week, I will not be available on Tuesdays. For urgent needs, please contact the office during regular hours."

That's it.

4. Enforce it. This is the hardest part. Because people will test it.

Patients will message you on Tuesday. Staff will call you with non-emergencies. Someone will say, "I know you're off, but can you just..."

The answer is no.

Not "I'll make an exception this one time." Not "Well, I guess I can help." No.

Because if you do not enforce the boundary, it is not a boundary. It is a suggestion.

And people will learn very quickly whether your boundaries are real or negotiable.

Dr. Kalli had to learn this the hard way. Dr. Kyle told her, "You cannot be on the premises. They will come find you."

And he was right. If she had stayed in the building on Tuesdays, staff would have knocked on her door. Patients would have asked for her. She would have gotten pulled back in.

So she left. She went home. She went to a coffee shop. She was physically unavailable. She muted her phone. She put it on Do Not Disturb.

And she read. She worked through *The Burnout Solution* chapter by chapter, taking notes, doing the exercises. She gave herself permission to just think, to breathe, to exist without being responsible for anyone else.

And the practice survived. More than survived—it thrived. Because the team learned to handle things without her.

Your first boundary will feel terrifying. Do it anyway.

Because every boundary you set makes the next one easier. And eventually, boundaries stop feeling like restrictions and start feeling like freedom.

What to Do Right Now (Your Stabilization Checklist)

If you are in acute burnout, here is what you do today:.

- **Acknowledge the crisis.** Stop pretending you are fine. You are not fine. That is okay. But you have to name it.
- **Notice your early warning signs.** Review the list earlier in this chapter. Which symptoms are you experiencing? Write them down.
- **Identify one boundary you can create this week.** Just one. What is the smallest change that would give you the most relief?
- **Communicate the boundary to one person.** Your spouse. Your office manager. A colleague. Say it out loud: "I need to change X."
- **Practice the 15-second reset.** Today. Between patients. Even if it feels ridiculous. Even if you are behind schedule.
- **Use the mantras.** When you feel yourself spiraling, stop. Breathe. Say, "I'm good. This is temporary."

- **Give yourself permission to ask for help.** If you need it. A therapist. A coach. A mentor. Someone who can help you stabilize.

This is not the end of the work. This is the beginning. But you have to stop the bleeding before you can heal the wound.

And you are stopping the bleeding right now.

What Comes Next

Stabilization is not recovery. It is triage.

You have stopped the acute crisis. You have created space to breathe. You have proven to yourself that change is possible. But you have not yet addressed the root cause.

And that is what we turn to next. In the next chapter, we are going to dismantle the lies you have been believing. We are going to show you how your perception—not your circumstances—is creating your burnout. Because once you understand that, you get your power back.

And that changes everything.

Reflection Questions:

1. What early warning signs have you been dismissing as "normal" that might actually be your body trying to get your attention?
2. If you could create one boundary this week that would give you immediate relief, what would it be?
3. What is stopping you from creating that boundary? (Be specific. Name the fear.)
4. What would it feel like to believe that your health is more important than one day's production?

CHAPTER 5

Root Causes: It Was Never Your Schedule

Dr. Kalli Hale had a revelation that changed everything. She was reading *The Burnout Solution*, taking notes, working through the exercises. She had blocked off Tuesdays. She was practicing the 15-second reset. She was using the mantras.

And the interventions were helping. She felt less frantic. Less reactive. More able to get through the day without feeling like she was drowning. But something deeper was shifting.

She read a chapter about how thoughts create your reality. About how the same circumstance can produce completely different emotional responses in people depending on how they perceived the threat.

Dr. Kalli had what she describes as a "light bulb moment."

The problem was not dentistry.

The problem was how she was <u>thinking</u> about dentistry.

The problem was not her schedule. It was how she was <u>interpreting</u> her schedule.

The problem was not difficult patients or demanding staff or tight finances. It was the meaning she was assigning to those things—the stories she was telling herself about what they meant regarding her future, her suffocation, her being trapped.

And once she understood that, everything changed.

Because if the problem was dentistry itself, there was only one solution: quit. But if the problem was her perception of dentistry, then there was another option: change the perception.

She could love dentistry again. She could build a sustainable practice. She could find joy in her work. Not by changing the external circumstances (though she would eventually do that too). But by changing how she thought about those circumstances.

This is the root cause, the deep work, what actually creates lasting change.

The Problem Isn't Dentistry (And Why That Changes Everything)

When you are burned out, it is easy to believe that the problem is the job itself.

Dentistry is too demanding. Dentistry is too stressful. Dentistry requires too much. If I could just get out of dentistry, everything would be better.

And for some people, that is true. Some people are genuinely in the wrong profession. They chose dentistry for the wrong reasons—family pressure, financial security, prestige—and they are miserable because they are doing work that does not align with who they are.

But that is not most burned-out dentists.

Most burned-out dentists actually love dentistry. Or they did, before burnout drained all the joy out of it. They love helping people. They love the precision of the work. They love solving clinical problems. They love building relationships with patients.

What they do not love is the way they have been practicing dentistry. The impossible schedule, the lack of boundaries, the financial pressure, the people-pleasing, the perfectionism, the constant anxiety about reviews and outcomes and whether they are doing enough.

That is not dentistry. That is how you have been doing dentistry.

Dr. Kalli was on the edge of quitting. But then she realized:

- The problem was that she had no boundaries, no systems, no protection from her own tendencies toward perfectionism and over-giving.
- The problem was that she was saying yes to everything and everyone, trying to be all things to all people, running herself into the ground trying to prove she was good enough.

- The problem was not the patients. It was that she had friended them all on Facebook and was answering their questions at 9 p.m.
- The problem was not the schedule. It was that she had no control over how she was being scheduled.
- The problem was not the staff. It was that she had gotten too close to one employee and created dysfunction in the team.

The problem was not dentistry. The problem was how she was doing dentistry.

And once she understood that, she had options. She did not have to quit. She had to redesign. And that changes everything.

Because if you believe the problem is dentistry, you feel trapped. Your only escape is to leave the profession entirely, which feels impossible when you have hundreds of thousands of dollars in student loans and a family to support.

But if you believe the problem is how you are practicing dentistry, you have power. You can make changes. You can set boundaries. You can build systems. You can redesign your practice so it supports you instead of draining you.

The first step in recovering from burnout is recognizing that the problem is not the job. It is how you are thinking about the job and how you are setting yourself up (or not setting yourself up) to do the job sustainably.

The Stress Equation (Demands > Resources)

Here is the formula for stress that most people do not understand:

Stress = Perceived Demands > Perceived Resources

Notice the word "perceived" in both parts of that equation.

Stress is not about *objective* reality. It is about your *subjective interpretation* of reality.

Two dentists can have the exact same schedule, the exact same patient load, the exact same circumstances—and one will be thriving while the other is burned out.

Why? Because they are perceiving those circumstances differently.

Dr. Kalli and her husband Dr. Kyle worked in the same practice. They saw similar numbers of patients. They dealt with similar cases. But Dr. Kyle was not burned out. Not because his circumstances were easier. But because he perceived them differently.

When a patient complained, Dr. Kyle thought, *Okay, let's solve this.* He did not personalize it. He did not catastrophize. He just saw it as a problem to fix.

When they got a one-star review, Dr. Kyle said, "Yeah, it sucks. You know what? We need to get 10 five-star reviews today. Y'all need to ask every single patient when they leave." He saw it as a numbers game. Not a referendum on his worth as a dentist.

When the schedule was packed, Dr. Kyle compartmentalized. He did the work, and then he went home and did not think about it again.

Dr. Kalli, on the other hand, took everything personally. A patient complaint meant she was failing. A one-star review meant she was a terrible dentist. A packed schedule meant she was trapped and would never escape.

Same circumstances. Different perceptions. Different outcomes.

Here is what this means practically:

You can reduce stress in two ways: reduce the demands or increase your resources.

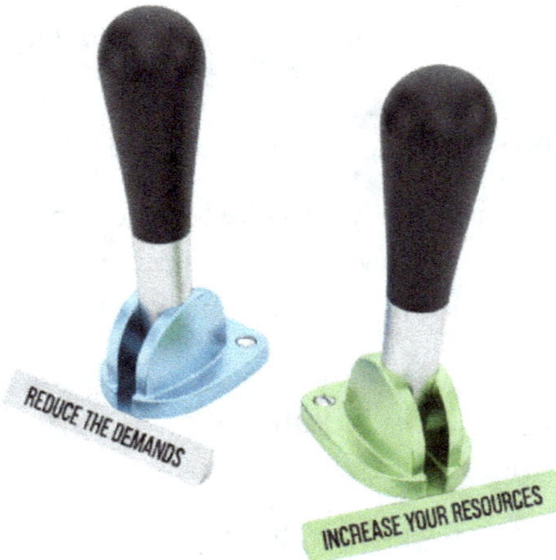

Most dentists only focus on the first option. They try to reduce the demands by seeing fewer patients, blocking more time, hiring more help.

And those things help. They are part of the solution. But they are not the whole solution. Because even with a perfectly designed schedule, you can still be stressed if you are perceiving the remaining demands as overwhelming.

You also have to work on the second part of the equation: increasing your perceived resources. And the fastest way to increase your perceived resources is to change how you think about the demands you face.

When you stop catastrophizing, you increase your resources.

When you stop personalizing, you increase your resources.

When you remind yourself that you have handled hard things before, you increase your resources.

When you recognize that most problems are temporary and solvable, you increase your resources.

This is not positive thinking. This is accurate thinking. And it is the difference between burning out and thriving.

What You're Making It Mean: The Crown the Patient Hates

Let's make this concrete.

You are in the operatory. You have just seated a crown. The patient looks in the mirror. And they say, "I don't like it." What happens next depends entirely on what you make that statement mean.

If you think it means: "I'm a terrible dentist. I did bad work. They're going to leave a one-star review and tell everyone I'm incompetent," then you are going to feel shame, anxiety, defensiveness. You are going to spiral. You might snap at the patient. You might obsess about it all night. You might question whether you are cut out for this profession.

If you think it means: "They have a different aesthetic preference than I anticipated. Let's figure out what they want and how we can adjust," then you are going to feel curious, collaborative, problem-solving. You are going to ask questions. You are going to work with the patient to find a solution. You might still feel some frustration, but you are not going to personalize it.

Same circumstance. Same patient statement. Completely different emotional response. And the difference is not what happened. The difference is what you made it mean.

Dr. Kalli describes this as one of the most powerful shifts from reading *The Burnout Solution*: "Maybe it's not all about *me*."

When a patient was upset, maybe they were just having a bad day. Maybe they were stressed about money. Maybe they were in pain and taking it out on her. Maybe they had unrealistic expectations that had nothing to do with the quality of her work.

It was not always about her.

But when you are burned out, everything feels personal. Every complaint is an indictment. Every problem is proof that you are failing. And that is exhausting.

Here is the practice: **When something stressful happens, pause and ask yourself, "What am I making this mean?"**

The patient is late. What are you making that mean? (Are you telling yourself they do not respect your time? Or are you recognizing that life is unpredictable and things happen?)

The staff member made a mistake. What are you making that mean? (Are you telling yourself they are incompetent and you cannot trust anyone? Or are you recognizing that mistakes happen and this is a training opportunity?)

Your production is down this month. What are you making that mean? (Are you telling yourself the practice is failing and you are a terrible business owner? Or are you recognizing that revenue fluctuates and this is one data point, not a trend?)

Most of the time, you are making things mean something catastrophic. Something personal. Something that reflects on your worth or competence. And that interpretation is what creates the stress. Not the circumstance itself. The meaning you assign to it.

Change the meaning, and you change the stress.

The Trap of Personalization: Boundaries, Betrayal, and Objectivity

One of the most common burnout triggers for dentists is taking patient complaints and staff conflicts personally. Whether it's an unhappy patient or a team member quitting, our instinct is to assume a personal failure: *I made a clinical error. I'm a bad leader. I failed them.*

While accountability is vital, the truth is that most of the time, **it is not about you.** People carry their own fears, financial stressors, and private baggage into your office. When you de-personalize these interactions, you create the mental space to respond thoughtfully instead of reacting defensively.

However, de-personalizing becomes nearly impossible when you blur the lines between "boss" and "best friend." Dr. Kalli learned this lesson the hard way through her relationship with her lead assistant, Katherine (not her real name).

Case Study: The Cost of Getting Too Close

In the early years of her practice, Dr. Kalli and Katherine were "thick as thieves." Dr. Kalli invested heavily in her, taking her to specialized trainings and relying on her as her right hand in complex airway cases. On the surface, they were a dream team.

But because Dr. Kalli had made Katherine her confidant, she lost her objectivity. She missed the growing dysfunction Katherine was creating within the rest of the team. Because she was "Kalli's girl," Katherine felt untouchable—refusing to help others and lording her status over the staff.

Dr. Kalli saw the red flags but ignored them. She was in the throes of burnout and terrified that if she confronted Katherine, she would lose her clinical support. By prioritizing the "friendship" over the leadership, she allowed the conflict to fester until one Thursday, Katherine quit abruptly with no warning.

The Lesson: Professional Distance is a Tool

Dr. Kalli felt completely betrayed, but that betrayal was a symptom of a missing boundary. When you get too close to an employee, you lose the ability to lead effectively. You cannot give honest feedback, you cannot enforce standards, and you inadvertently breed resentment among the rest of the team who see the favoritism.

When Katherine tried to return a year later, Dr. Kalli remembered her father's advice: *"Once you fire someone—or they walk away—don't fall for the excuses to bring them back."* She said no, knowing that rehiring her would only recreate the same toxic environment.

The Practice for Maintaining Perspective

To avoid the burnout that comes from these emotional rollercoasters, you must practice both **internal de-personalization** and **external boundaries**:

- **Ask the "What Else" Question:** When a patient or staff member is upset, ask: *"What else could this be about?"* Are they facing financial pressure? A sick child? Burnout of their own? This shifts the focus from your perceived "failure" to the reality of their circumstances.
- **Warmth vs. Intimacy:** Be warm and show your team you care, but maintain a professional distance. Do not share things with one employee that you wouldn't share with the whole team.

- **Lead Through Discomfort:** Do not avoid difficult conversations about performance or fit because you are afraid of hurting someone's feelings.

You can take responsibility for your part and apologize when appropriate, but you do not have to carry the weight of believing every problem is your fault. When you prioritize being "liked" over running your business well, everyone—including you—suffers.

Fusion vs. Differentiation: Your Identity Beyond the Practice

There is a concept in psychology called "differentiation of self." It means having a clear sense of who you are—your values, your boundaries, your identity—that is separate from the people around you.

When you are poorly differentiated, you are "fused" with others. Their emotions become your emotions. Their approval becomes your worth. Their problems become your responsibility.

And this is a massive problem for dentists. Because you are trained to be responsible. You are trained to fix problems. You are trained to meet needs.

So when a patient is unhappy, you feel responsible for their happiness. When a staff member is struggling, you feel responsible for fixing it. When your practice is not perfect, you feel like a failure.

You are fused with your practice. Your identity is completely wrapped up in being a dentist, being a practice owner, being the person who takes care of everyone.

And when you are that fused, you have no buffer. No protection. Every problem in the practice feels like a personal attack. Every setback feels like proof that you are not good enough.

Dr. Kalli was completely fused with her practice. When Katherine quit, it felt like a personal betrayal—not a business decision, but a relationship betrayal. When a patient was unhappy, it felt like Dr. Kalli had failed as a person, not just as a clinician. When production was down, it felt like Dr. Kalli was worthless, not just that the practice had a slow month. She could not separate herself from the practice. They were one and the same in her mind. And that is suffocating.

Here is what differentiation looks like:

You care deeply about your work without making your work the measure of your worth.

You can have a bad day at the practice and still know you are a good person.

You can have a patient leave a one-star review and still know you are a competent dentist.

You can have an employee quit and still know you are a good leader.

Because your identity is not dependent on any single outcome. You are not your production numbers. You are not your patient satisfaction scores. You are not your staff retention rate.

You are a human being with inherent worth. And the work you do—while important—is not what makes you valuable. This is deep work. It does not happen overnight. But it starts with recognizing when you are fused.

When you find yourself spiraling because a patient was unhappy, pause. Ask yourself: "Am I making this about my worth as a person? Or can I see this as a business problem to solve?"

When a staff member quits and you feel devastated, pause. Ask yourself: "Am I taking this personally? Or can I recognize that people make decisions for their own reasons that have nothing to do with me?"

Differentiation does not mean you stop caring. It means you care without losing yourself in the process.

The Cost of Caring: Navigating Compassion Fatigue

In the world of healthcare, we often praise the "infinite well" of service—the idea that a truly dedicated professional should be able to give endlessly to their patients. But there is a biological and emotional reality that contradicts this: **Compassion is a finite resource.**

Think of your emotional capacity like a **reservoir**. In a healthy practice, the water flows out to provide for your patients, but it is also replenished by rest, boundaries, and professional satisfaction. Compassion fatigue occurs when the outflow is so aggressive, and the walls of the reservoir so porous, that the water level drops until you are scraping the dry, cracked earth at the bottom.

Burnout vs. Compassion Fatigue

While they often travel together, it is important to distinguish between the two. **Burnout** is the exhaustion resulting from chronic workplace stress—the "grind" of the schedule, the paperwork, and the overhead. **Compassion fatigue**, however, is the emotional saturation that comes from caring too much without a filter. It is the "cost of caring."

When you suffer from compassion fatigue, you aren't just tired of the work; you are depleted by the *people*. It manifests as:

- **Emotional Numbness:** Feeling detached or "robbed" of your ability to care.
- **Empathy Failure:** Struggling to feel compassion even when you know a patient is suffering.
- **Resentment:** Feeling a quiet anger toward patients for having needs or "taking" from you.
- **The "Going Through the Motions" Syndrome:** Dr. Kalli describes this as losing her heart for the patient experience—performing the clinical tasks perfectly while being completely absent emotionally.

The Irony of the Healer

The cruel irony of dentistry is that the very traits that make you an excellent clinician—your empathy, your desire to alleviate pain, and your high standards—are the exact traits that make you vulnerable to this depletion. If you view your role as being a "human shield" for your patients' fears and discomforts, you will eventually reach a point of emotional bankruptcy.

The Shift: Caring Sustainably

To move from a state of depletion back to a state of overflow, you must shift your perspective on what "good care" looks like.

- **Responsibility vs. Support:** You are responsible *to* your patients (for providing excellent clinical care), but you are not responsible *for* them (for their lifelong habits, their emotional reactions, or their personal choices).
- **Empathy vs. Absorption:** You can acknowledge a patient's fear without taking that fear home with you. You can witness their pain without making it your own.
- **The "Oxygen Mask" Principle:** It is a cliché for a reason—you cannot pour from an empty cup. If you drain your reservoir to the point of a drought, you become useless to the very people you want to help.

The goal is to remain a vibrant, healthy source of care—strong and rooted—while understanding that you must protect your "water level." Setting a limit on what you give isn't an act of selfishness; it is the only way to ensure you have something left to give tomorrow.

The Math That Puts It in Perspective (1 Out of 3,000)

Here is an exercise that helps de-catastrophize negative reviews and patient complaints.

When you get a one-star review or a patient complains, ask yourself:

How many patients have I seen this year?

Let's say you see 15 new patients a month. That is 180 new patients a year. Plus your existing patient base of, let's say, 1,500 active patients.

So you are interacting with roughly 1,700 to 2,000 patients in a given year.

Now ask yourself:

How many of those patients were unhappy enough to complain or leave a bad review?

Maybe one. Maybe two. Maybe five in a really bad year.

Now do the math. If one patient out of 2,000 left a one-star review, what percentage of your patients does that represent?

0.05%.

That means 99.95% of your patients did not feel compelled to leave a negative review.

But you are spending hours—maybe days—obsessing over that one person. That 0.05%. And you are ignoring the 99.95% who were fine. Who were happy. Who had a good experience.

This is the negativity bias of the brain. We are wired to focus on threats, on problems, on things that go wrong. Because evolutionarily, that kept us alive. But in modern life, it makes us miserable.

One negative review gets more mental real estate than 100 positive interactions. One patient complaint weighs heavier than 1,000 patients who were satisfied.

You need to consciously counteract that bias with data.

When you get a negative review, do not spiral. Do the math.

How many patients did I serve? How many were happy? What is the actual percentage this represents?

And then remind yourself: **This is one data point. It does not define me. It does not define my practice.**

You can learn from it if there is something legitimate to learn. You can make changes if changes are warranted. But you do not have to let it destroy you. Because one unhappy patient out of 2,000 is not evidence that you are a terrible dentist. It is evidence that you are human, and not everyone will be pleased all the time. And that is okay.

What This All Means

Here is the core message of this chapter:

Burnout is not caused by your circumstances. It is caused by how you think about and handle your circumstances.

Yes, you may need to change your schedule. Yes, you may need to set boundaries. Yes, you may need to hire help or get out of network with insurance. But those external changes will not stick if you do not also change your internal narrative.

Because you can have a perfect schedule and still be burned out if you are catastrophizing every challenge. You can have great staff and still be miserable if you are taking every issue personally. You can have thriving production and still feel empty if your worth is tied to external validation.

The root cause of burnout is not the demands of dentistry. It is the way you perceive those demands and the meaning you assign to them. And that is actually good news. Because while you cannot always control your circumstances, you can control your perception.

You can choose to stop personalizing.

You can choose to stop catastrophizing.

You can choose to separate your worth from your productivity.

You can choose to see problems as solvable instead of evidence of your failure.

This is the work we do in coaching together. This is what creates lasting change.

Not only rearranging your schedule. But rearranging how you think about your schedule. Not only setting boundaries. But changing the beliefs that made you afraid to set boundaries in the first place. Not only surviving dentistry. But learning to thrive in it.

And that is what the next section is about: building the systems—both internal and external—that allow you to practice dentistry in a way that is sustainable, fulfilling, and aligned with the life you actually want to live.

Reflection Questions:

1. What is one recurring stressor in your practice that you have been personalizing? How would your experience change if you de-personalized it?
2. When was the last time you felt fused with your practice—unable to separate your worth from your work? What would differentiation look like for you?
3. Think of a recent patient complaint or negative review. What percentage of your total patient interactions does it represent? Does that change how you feel about it?
4. Where are you giving like The Giving Tree—giving until you are a stump? What boundary would allow you to keep giving sustainably?

CHAPTER 6

From Financial Quicksand To Control

Dr. Kalli Hale remembers the day she realized that her clinical excellence was being subsidized by her own exhaustion.

She was seeing 140 new patients a month, sprinting through four-day weeks in an attempt to provide an elite experience. But the math of the "insurance grind" was a trap. When she finally sat down to calculate the gap between what insurance paid and the actual cost of the high-touch care she refused to compromise on, the numbers were devastating.

She wasn't just working hard; she was paying for the privilege of treating her patients.

A single cleaning or a standard filling barely covered the overhead of the materials and the talented team she had assembled. She was running on a treadmill that kept getting faster, yet she remained financially stationary. The insurance companies held the remote—dictating terms, delaying payments, and demanding justifications for her clinical decisions.

Dr. Kalli felt suffocated. It was in that moment of "financial quicksand" that she made a decision that terrified her: **She was going to reclaim her practice.**

She didn't do it all at once; she couldn't afford to. Instead, she began systematically resigning from the "worst offender" networks. She stopped trying to be everything to every insurance provider and started focusing on her "patient avatar"—the ideal patient who valued five-star care and a community-focused experience over a co-pay.

The transition took two years. It was a period defined by constant communication, the fear of making a catastrophic mistake, and the hope that her patients would see the value in her independence. But it was the decision that saved her.

Once she was out-of-network, the "grind" began to dissolve. She regained the power to set her own fees, design a human-centric schedule, and invest time where it actually mattered. She discovered a hard truth: **Financial freedom and mental freedom are inseparable.**

You cannot recover from burnout while you are a hostage to someone else's fee schedule. When you are dependent on volume to outrun low reimbursements, you lose the ability to say "no." But when you take control of the finances, you take back your life.

The patients she feared losing? Most of them stayed. They didn't just want a dentist; they wanted *her* care. As her revenue stabilized, her burnout began to lift. This chapter is about how to stop drowning in the quotas and start building the firm financial foundation required for a sustainable career.

The Diminishing Returns of Overwork

Let's start with a hard truth that most dentists do not want to hear.

Working more hours does not necessarily make you more money.

In fact, past a certain point, working more hours makes you less productive, less effective, and more likely to burn out.

Remember the research we discussed in Chapter 2? Pencavel's 2014 study from Stanford showed that productivity per hour declines sharply when the work week exceeds 50 hours. And after 55 hours, productivity drops so precipitously that someone working 70 hours produces little more than someone working 55 hours.

The extra 15 hours are essentially wasted effort. You are there physically, but you are not operating at full capacity. You are making more mistakes. You are moving slower. You are less focused.

And in dentistry, where precision matters and errors have consequences, working when you are mentally and physically depleted is not just inefficient—it is dangerous.

But here is the trap most dentists fall into:

You graduate with $300,000 in debt. You need to start making money immediately. So you work as much as you can. You say yes to every opportunity. You pack your schedule. You stay late. You take emergency calls on the weekends.

And it works. For a while. You start paying down debt. You build a patient base. The practice grows. But you also build habits that are unsustainable. You train yourself to equate hours worked with income earned. You start to believe that the only way to make more money is to work more hours. And you get stuck on the hamster wheel.

When Dr. Kyle forced Dr. Kalli to cut Tuesdays, she was convinced it wasn't feasible. But here is what actually happened:

Her production did not drop 25%. It dropped maybe 10%. Because the other three days, she was more focused. More efficient. Less exhausted. She made fewer mistakes. She had better patient interactions. Her case acceptance went up because she was not rushing through consultations. Her teams also worked hard to learn how to schedule her better, make the time she was there extremely productive, while she trained her assistants to help with the tasks she did NOT need to be in the operatory for! And then, when she hired associate dentists to cover some of the load, her overall practice production went *up* even though she was working *fewer* hours.

Because she stopped being the bottleneck.

Here is the principle: **Past a certain point, working more hours is not the solution. Working smarter is.**

And working smarter means:

- Designing a schedule that allows you to operate at peak capacity instead of constant depletion
- Delegating tasks that do not require your clinical expertise
- Train your RDA's to be a extension of YOU
- Hiring help so you are not the only producer in the practice
- Setting fees that actually compensate you fairly for your time and expertise

- Saying no to low-value work (like insurance that reimburses at rates below your costs)

You cannot out-hustle burnout. You can only out-think it.

Getting Out of Network: Dr. Kalli's Two-Year Battle

Getting out of network with insurance is one of the most terrifying decisions a dentist can make. Because you are essentially betting that patients will value your care enough to pay out of pocket or accept lower reimbursement from out-of-network benefits. And if you are wrong, you could lose a significant portion of your patient base.

Dr. Kalli knew this. She agonized over it. She delayed as long as she could. But eventually, the math forced her hand.

She ran a report on the lowest-reimbursing insurance she was in-network with. She calculated exactly how much they were paying versus how much it cost to deliver that care. And she realized: **She literally could not afford to provide the elite care she intended to...AND stay in network with this insurance.**

So she made the decision. She was dropping it. But she did not do it recklessly. She had a strategy.

Step 1: Communicate early and clearly.

She gave patients six months' notice. Her front desk staff called every patient who had that insurance and explained: "Dr. Hale is going out of network with [Insurance Company] effective [Date]. You will still be able to see us, and we will still file claims for you, but the reimbursement may be different. We wanted you to know ahead of time so you can make the best decision for your family."

Some patients left. Dr. Kalli was prepared for that. But most stayed. Because they had been seeing her for years. They trusted her. They valued the care. *The ones that stayed were the patients she truly wanted anyway.*

Step 2: Honor the reimbursement for preventive care during the transition.

Here is the brilliant part. For the first year after going out of network, Dr. Kalli continued to honor the in-network reimbursement rate for cleanings and preventive care.

Why? Because most patients do not know the cost of fillings or crowns off the top of their head. But they know they were getting their cleanings for "free". So she told patients, "We're going out of network, but for one year—i will still honor the in-network fee for your cleanings And patients thought, *Okay, that's not so bad. I don't have to find a new dentist for my cleaning RIGHT NOW.*

But for everything else—fillings, crowns, root canals—she could charge her actual fees. And patients did not push back because they did not have the same reference point. Patients don't really WANT to change their dentist anyway!

This strategy allowed her to transition out of network without losing her hygiene patients as quickly

Step 3: Identify the next insurance to drop.

Once she successfully dropped the first one, she did it again. And again. Over two years, she systematically got out of network with every insurance company that was not worth the reimbursement.

And here is what happened: **Her stress went down. Her income went up. And her schedule became manageable.**

Because she was no longer seeing patients just to hit volume targets for insurance. She was seeing the patients she actually wanted to serve, at fees that actually compensated her fairly. She also had happier hygienists, because she could give them a full 90 minutes for a new patient exam, a full 60 minutes for a recall appointment, and an hour per quad for SRP's. She actually told the hygienists to tell HER how much time they wanted - then, she made it happen.

Getting out of network is not for everyone. But if you are in-network and burned out, you need to at least run the numbers.

Calculate what insurance is actually paying you. Factor in the time, the materials, the overhead, the stress of dealing with claims and denials.

And ask yourself: **Is this worth it?**

If the answer is no, you have options. You do not have to stay trapped.

The Patient Avatar: Who Do You Actually Want to Serve?

Here is a question most dentists never ask themselves:

Who is my ideal patient?

Not "Who can afford to pay?" Not "Who has good insurance?" But: **Who do I actually want to serve?**

Dr. Kalli did not think about this until years into practice. She just assumed she had to treat everyone. Anyone with teeth and a pulse. But then she started taking courses in biologic dentistry. She was learning about materials, about the systemic impacts of oral health, about airway and sleep and whole-body wellness.

And she realized: the patients who were most excited about this kind of care were not the ones coming in for their "free insurance cleaning".

They were the patients who cared about their health, who asked questions, who valued prevention, who were willing to invest in long-term wellness instead of just fixing problems when they broke.

Those were the patients who energized her, the cases she loved, the interactions that made her remember why she became a dentist.

And the patients who just wanted the cheapest, fastest fix? They were draining. They did not value her expertise. They fought her on treatment recommendations. They left bad reviews when things did not go perfectly.

So Dr. Kalli made a decision: **She was going to design her practice around her ideal patient.**

Here is the exercise that changed everything for her:

Describe your ideal patient in detail.

Not just demographics. But values, priorities, and attitudes.

For Dr. Kalli, her ideal patient:

- Values health and prevention over just fixing problems
- Asks questions and wants to understand their treatment
- Is willing to invest in quality care
- Respects her time and expertise
- Has a positive, collaborative attitude

Once she had clarity on that, she could make decisions accordingly.

She could market to that type of patient instead of trying to appeal to everyone.

She could design her services around what those patients valued.

She could set fees that reflected the level of care she wanted to provide.

And she could let go of patients who were not a good fit—without guilt.

Because here is the truth: **You cannot and should not serve everyone.**

If you try to be everything to everyone, you end up burned out and resentful.

But if you get clear on who you are meant to serve, you can build a practice that attracts the right people and repels the wrong ones.

Your practice is not a public utility. You do not have to accept every patient who calls.

You get to choose. And that choice is one of the most powerful tools you have for preventing burnout and looking forward to the patients on your schedule

Ideal Scheduling vs. the Overbooked Nightmare

Let's talk about the schedule. Your schedule is either your greatest tool for sustainability or your biggest source of stress. Most dentists have the second kind.

They are overbooked. Back-to-back patients. No buffer time. No lunch. No bathroom breaks. Double-booked columns because the front desk is trying to squeeze in "just one more." They tell themselves, *This is just what it takes. If I want to make money, I have to stay busy.*

But here is what Dr. Kalli learned: **Being busy is not the same as being productive.**

When you are overbooked, you are constantly running behind. You are rushing through appointments. You are making mistakes. You are providing lower-quality care. You are stressed and irritable.

And your patients feel it. They can tell you are rushed. They can sense your stress. And that affects their experience.

Ideal scheduling is the opposite. It is about designing your schedule so that you have enough time to do excellent work without feeling frantic.

Here is what that looks like in practice:
1. Build in buffer time.

Dr. Kalli learned this from her husband, Dr. Kyle, and from redesigning her practice after burnout. She stopped scheduling patients in a way that left no room for the unexpected. Instead, she gave herself cushion. If a procedure typically took 30 minutes, she blocked 45. If it typically took an hour, she blocked 75 minutes.

Why? Because things happen. The patient is late. The case is more complex than anticipated. You need a minute to think or to call a specialist or to just breathe. If you schedule everything at the absolute minimum time required, you have zero margin for error. And dentistry always has variables. But if you build in buffer time, you can handle the unexpected without everything falling apart.

2. Block time for non-clinical work.

You are not just a clinician. You are also a business owner (or an employee managing your own career). You need time to review cases, call specialists, handle administrative tasks, train staff, work on marketing, check your financials. If you do not block time for that during the workday, you end up doing it at night and on weekends. Which means you never stop working. Dr. Kalli blocked Tuesdays for business work. That was non-negotiable time for her to catch up on things that did not require being in the operatory.

3. Honor your lunch break.

This sounds obvious. But most dentists skip lunch. Dr. Kalli did. For years. She would just grab a protein bar between patients and keep going. But when you do not eat, your blood sugar crashes. Your focus deteriorates. Your mood tanks. You make worse decisions. A 30-minute lunch break is not optional. It is essential for maintaining performance. Block it on your schedule. Make it sacred. Leave the building if you have to.

4. Stop double-booking yourself.

This is where most dentists lose control of their schedule. The front desk sees an opening and thinks, *We can squeeze this patient in.* So they double-book you without asking. And suddenly you are supposed to be in two places at once. Dr. Kalli had to have a hard conversation with her team: "You do not get to double-book me without my permission. If someone needs to be squeezed in, you ask me first. And if I say no, the answer is no." This felt harsh at first. But it was necessary. Because your team does not experience the stress of a double-booked schedule the way you do. They are trying to help. They are trying to accommodate patients. But they are also creating chaos. You have to take control.

5. Design around your energy, not just your availability.

Not all hours are created equal. You might be most focused and energetic in the morning. So schedule your most complex cases then. You might hit a slump after lunch. So schedule easier appointments then. You might be completely depleted by 4 p.m. So stop scheduling patients after 3. Work with your natural rhythms instead of fighting them.

6. Design your second column for a highly trained RDA

You can only be in one room at a time.

To help with that, Dr. Kalli separated her schedule into a high-production primary column and an assistant-led side column for non-production tasks (like crown seats or Invisalign checks). Her treatment coordinators had to learn how to schedule those columns so Dr. Kalli could be put to use in the most productive way possible. This also meant coordinating the hygiene schedule appropriately so it flowed well with the doctor columns.

Scheduling is an art: ensure your staff is fully trained and that patients are informed ahead of time whether they will be seeing the doctor or the assistant.

The Bottom Line

Ideal scheduling is not about seeing fewer patients. It is about seeing patients in a way that allows you to do your best work without destroying yourself.

When you shift from a reactive schedule to an intentional one, something remarkable happens: **your production stays the same, or even increases, while your stress evaporates.** You finally stop operating from a state of constant depletion and start working at peak capacity.

The Cushion Strategy That Prevents Chaos

Here is the secret to sustainable scheduling: **Always give yourself more time than you think you need.**

According to Dr. Kalli, "If a patient appointment only needs 15 minutes, book it for 30 minutes. You need wiggle room within your day for unexpected appointments or to sit at your desk for a second, write some notes, etc."

This is the cushion strategy. You are not padding the schedule to charge them more. You are building in margin for the unexpected. Because dentistry is full of the unexpected.

If you have scheduled everything at the bare minimum, any deviation creates a cascade of delays. You get behind. You start rushing. You get stressed. The rest of the day suffers.

And here is the bonus: on the days when everything goes smoothly, you get time back. Time to sit down. Time to think. Time to decompress between patients. That is not wasted time. That is recovery time. And it is what allows you to sustain high performance instead of burning out.

The cushion strategy is how you go from feeling like a victim of your schedule to feeling like you control your schedule.

Multiple Income Streams Beyond the Chair

There is a limiting belief that keeps many dentists trapped: *The only way to make money is to be the one holding the drill.*

For years, this was Dr. Kalli's reality. Her personal production was over a million dollars a year, but it was entirely clinical. If she wasn't in the operatory, the revenue stopped. She was trapped by her own success—unable to reduce her hours or take an extended vacation without a devastating hit to her income.

She realized she needed to move from trading "time for money" to building a practice that worked for *her*. This is the concept of **leverage**: creating systems or assets that produce income without requiring your direct, hands-on labor.

The Mindset of Multipliers

The first step toward leverage is a fundamental mindset shift regarding your team.

- **The Old Thought:** "If I hire an associate, I'll make less money because I have to pay them."
- **The Leverage Thought:** "If I hire an associate, I am buying back my time and increasing the practice's total capacity."

As Dr. Kalli puts it: *"I realized I could consciously cut another day from my week, knowing the practice was going to be okay because I had two other full-time dentists producing."* By sharing a percentage of the revenue, she gained something far more valuable: her sanity and the freedom to pick her kids up from school every day.

Diversifying the Income Stream

Once Dr. Kalli mastered leverage within the office, she began to see possibilities beyond the four walls of the clinic. Today, her income is no longer dependent on her own clinical hours. Her portfolio of leverage includes:

- **Group Practice Ownership:** With 10+ locations, she has created a stellar patient experience that scales. She cannot be in ten places at once, but her systems can.
- **Educational Assets:** She turned her expertise into a teledentistry company and recorded courses on patient experience. She created these once, and they now serve others indefinitely.
- **Mentorship & Consulting:** She is now paid for her *expertise* and her *vision*, not just her manual dexterity.
- **Strategic Reinvestment:** Using practice profits to invest in real estate, opening more practices, ensuring her money works as hard as she once did.

Freedom is About Choices

The goal of creating multiple income streams isn't necessarily to quit clinical dentistry—it's to make clinical dentistry **optional**.

Financial freedom isn't a specific number in a bank account; it is the ability to choose. If you want to cut back to two days a week, you can. If you want to focus on teaching, you can. The more streams of income you build, the more choices you have, and the further you move away from the "financial quicksand" of burnout.

The Associate's Survival Guide: Control Without Ownership

Not everyone wants to own a practice. And that is okay.

If you are an associate dentist, you face different challenges. You do not have control over the schedule. You do not set the fees. You do not decide what insurance to accept. You do not hire or fire staff. Someone else makes those decisions. And if they make bad decisions, you are the one who suffers.

Dr. Kalli has worked with many burned-out associates. And the number one complaint she hears is: **long hours and lack of control.**

They feel like the schedule controls them. Like they have to stay until 6 p.m. even though they want to leave at 3 p.m. Like they cannot make decisions about their own patients. And that lack of autonomy is a major burnout driver.

Here is what Dr. Kalli tells associates who are struggling: **You have more power than you think. But you have to use it.** Most associates do not negotiate. They accept the terms they are given. They assume they have to just deal with whatever the practice owner decides.

But here is the truth: **Good associates are hard to find. And practices do not want to lose you.** As an associate, you are making money for the business. If you quit, they have to find someone else. Train someone else. Deal with the communication with the patients that you have left. That is a huge pain for them. So you have leverage. You just have to use it.

How to have the conversation:

If you are burned out as an associate, do not just quit. Have a conversation with the practice owner.

Sit down with them and say:

"I love working here. I want to stay. But I need to make some changes to my schedule [or my patient load, or my working hours] in order to sustain this long-term. Can we talk about what that might look like?"

Be specific. Do not say, "I'm stressed." Say, "I need to leave at 3 p.m. on Fridays so I can pick my kids up from school."

Or, "I need one afternoon a week blocked off for non-clinical work."

Or, "I need to stop seeing patients after 5 p.m. because I'm exhausted by the end of the day."

Most practice owners will work with you. Because they do not want to lose you. But you have to ask. You have to advocate for yourself. And if you ask and they say no—if they are unwilling to make any accommodations to help you avoid burnout—then you know: **this is not the right place for you.** And you have permission to leave.

Dr. Kalli is very clear about what she offers her associates: "I decided if that became something in our large practice group I would do my best to honor their request— I would work like heck to get a second provider in there that maybe only wanted to work afternoons, who knows, so that we could have the best of both worlds. And I know that I will keep my doctors much longer than your traditional chain dental office."

She is intentional about creating an environment where associates do not burn out. Because she has been there. She knows what it feels like.

If you are an associate, find a practice owner who values your wellbeing. And if you are a practice owner, create an environment where your associates can thrive. Because turnover is expensive. Burnout is expensive. And investing in your personal sustainability is one of the smartest business decisions you can make.

From Quicksand to Solid Ground

Financial stress and burnout are deeply interconnected.

When you feel financially trapped—whether because of debt, insurance dependency, or feeling like you have to see every patient just to make ends meet—you cannot make the changes necessary to recover from burnout.

But when you take control of your finances, everything shifts.

You can say no to insurance that does not serve you.

You can design a schedule that supports your wellbeing instead of maxing out your capacity.

You can build multiple income streams so you are not dependent on clinical production alone.

You can hire help and create leverage so you are not doing everything yourself.

Financial freedom and mental freedom go hand in hand.

And the path from quicksand to solid ground starts with one decision: **I am going to run my practice (or my career) in a way that serves me, not just my bottom line.**

For Dr. Kalli, that decision looked like getting out of network, even though it felt risky. It looked like hiring associates, even though it meant giving up production. It looked like blocking time off her schedule, even though she was convinced she could not afford it. Every decision felt risky. Every change felt scary. But each one brought her closer to the practice—and the life—she actually wanted. And that is what we are building toward: not just surviving dentistry, but thriving in it.

The next chapter is where we get tactical. We are going to talk about the systems—the actual processes and protocols—that Dr. Kalli built to prevent burnout and create a practice that runs smoothly even when she is not there.

Because mindset shifts are essential. Financial control is essential. But *systems* are what make it all stick.

Reflection Questions:

1. If you ran the numbers, what would you discover about your insurance reimbursements versus your actual costs? Are you making money or losing money on certain procedures?
2. Who is your ideal patient? Describe them in detail. How would your practice change if you designed it around serving that person?
3. Where is your schedule controlling you instead of you controlling it? What is one change you could make this week to create more margin?
4. If you are an associate: What is the one thing you most need to change about your working conditions? Have you asked for it? If not, what is stopping you?
5. What would financial freedom look like for you? What income streams beyond clinical dentistry could you explore?

PART III

Restoration & Fortification

CHAPTER 7

The Systems That Save You: The Patient First Framework By Sleep Well™

Dr. Kalli Hale stood on a stage in Chicago, speaking to a room full of dentists.

She was not there to teach clinical techniques. She was not demonstrating how to place an implant or prep a crown. She was there because someone had asked her a question she had never really considered: **"Why are you so good at what you do?"**

Not just clinically. But holistically. Why did her practice thrive? Why did patients stay? Why did her team function well? Why, after recovering from severe burnout, was she now running multiple successful practices while also picking her kids up from school every day?

She had to think about it. Because when you are in the thick of building something, you do not always see the system you have created. You just do what works.

But as she prepared for that presentation, she realized: **She had built a system. A very specific, very intentional system for the entire patient journey—from the first phone call to the final follow-up.**

And that system was not just good for patients. It was good for her. Because when you have systems, you do not have to make everything up as you go. You do not have to hold everything in your head. You do not have to be the only person who knows how things work.

Systems create predictability. Consistency. Ease.

And for a burned-out dentist trying to regain control of her practice, systems were the difference between drowning and thriving.

This is what she came to call **The Patient First Framework by Sleep Well™.** And it is what we are going to unpack in this chapter.

Because the right systems do not just improve patient satisfaction. They prevent burnout.

Start With the End in Mind: Designing for Sustainability

Most dentists do not design their practices. They inherit processes from wherever they trained or worked before. They do things "the way they have always been done."

And then they wonder why they feel frantic, disorganized, and burned out.

Dr. Kalli learned this lesson the hard way. In the early years, she was reactive. A patient called, and the front desk scheduled them however they could fit. A patient arrived, and the team scrambled to figure out who would take them back. A case needed follow-up, and it either happened or entirely forgotten, because of lack of systems.

The lack of systems reared their ugly head as her practice became more and more successful. Her parents used the phrase "when you get busy, that's when the wheels fall off…" to encourage her to create better systems.

So when Dr. Kalli started to rebuild after burnout, she asked herself a different question:

What kind of day do I want to have when I'm at work?

Not just financially or clinically, but experientially.

What do I want it to feel like to work here? What do I want patients to experience? What do I want my team to be able to do without constantly asking me for direction?

And then she designed backward from that vision.

She wanted patients to feel cared for from the moment they called. She wanted her team to feel confident and empowered. She wanted herself to walk into an operatory knowing exactly what was happening and why, without having to ask a hundred questions. So she built systems to create that experience.

Here is the principle: **Systems are not about rigidity. They are about freedom.**

When you have a system for how the phone should be answered, your front desk does not have to guess. They know what to say. They feel confident.

When you have a system for how patients move from the waiting room to the operatory, your assistants and hygienists do not have to improvise. They know the process. It happens smoothly.

When you have a system for treatment handoffs and follow-ups, things do not fall through the cracks. Patients get the care they need. You do not lie awake at night wondering if you forgot to call someone.

Your systems will also save your life when it comes to replacing employees.

Systems take the mental load off you. And that is how they prevent burnout.

The Phone-to-Follow-Up Pathway That Prevents Burnout

Dr. Kalli built a visual framework that maps the entire patient journey. It starts with the first phone call and ends with follow-up after treatment.

Every touchpoint is intentional. Every interaction is designed. Nothing is left to chance.

Here is the pathway:

1. The First Phone Call
2. Waiting Room Experience
3. Retrieval to Operatory
4. Operatory Setup
5. Intake and Co-Diagnosis
6. Doctor Experience
7. Treatment Coordination and Handoff
8. Exit Experience

9. Post-Op Calls

10. Review Requests

11. Follow-Up Cadence

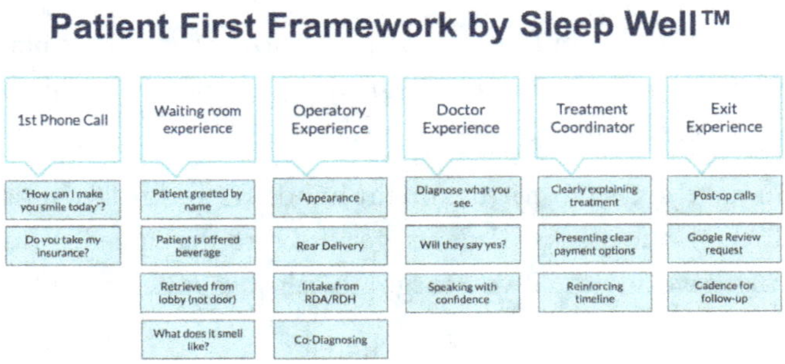

Each of these touchpoints has a system, a script, a protocol, a way it should be done.

And when everyone on the team knows the system, the practice runs smoothly. Patients have a great experience. And the dentist is not constantly putting out fires or making everything up on the fly.

Let's walk through each step.

"How Can I Make You Smile Today?": Scripts That Work

The first impression a patient has of your practice is the phone call. And most dental offices blow it.

The phone rings. Someone answers, distracted, mid-conversation with someone else in the office. "Thank you for calling New Teeth Dental Solutions, can you please hold?".

Or they answer with no energy, no warmth, just going through the motions. "New Teeth Dental Solutions, how can I help you?"

This is not good enough.

Dr. Kalli decided that every phone call should start with a smile. Literally.

She put a mirror on the front desk. And she told her team: **When you answer the phone, look in the mirror and make sure you are smiling.**

Why? Because people can hear a smile through the phone. Your voice changes when you smile. It sounds warmer, more welcoming, more alive.

And she gave them a script:

"Thank you for calling New Teeth Dental Solutions! How can I make you smile today?"

It is different. It is memorable. It sets a tone. And here is what happens: patients respond. They laugh. They relax. They feel like they called a place that actually cares about them.

But the script does not stop there. Because the next question is usually about insurance. And this is where most practices lose that patient opportunity. You must curate the response you want your team to say in response to these questions!

The caller asks, "Do you take [xxx] insurance?" and your team responds with "No, I'm sorry, we don't." The call will end with an "okay, thank you, bye."

That is a lost patient. A lost opportunity. A lost chance at edifying the practice, the team, and the doctor to convince a patient you are worth the extra money.

Dr. Kalli trained her team differently.

When a patient asks about insurance, here is what they say:

"I'd love to check that for you. We are not technically in-network with any plans based on the elite services we provide here at New Teeth - but let me see what your out-of-network benefits might cover. We would love to treat you and your family. Dr. Kalli has been doing this a long time, and you will love our office."

Notice what that does:

- It does not shut the conversation down
- It offers to help (looking up benefits)
- It sets an expectation (might be surprised)
- It builds value (Dr. Kalli has experience, you will love the office)

You are not begging. You are not apologizing. You are just being helpful and confident.

And most of the time, patients stay on the line. They book the appointment. They come in.

The script matters. Train your team on exactly what to say. And then audit your calls to make sure they are saying it. Dr. Kalli uses a phone service that records calls. And she spot-checks them.

If you aren't checking these recordings, you have no idea what's being said on the other line.

Having scripts allows you to hold your team accountable for how you expect the calls to be answered. If they stop doing it the way you want: retrain. Remind them. Role-plays with them.

Because the phone call is where it all starts. If you lose patients there, you never get a chance to deliver great care.

The Waiting Room Experience (Including What It Smells Like)

The patient books an appointment. They show up. They walk through the door. What happens next?

In most dental offices, the patient walks in and nobody looks up. The front desk is busy on the computer or on the phone. The patient stands there awkwardly. Maybe there is a clipboard on a shelf with a sign that says, "Please sign in." This is terrible.

Dr. Kalli's practice does it differently.

Every patient is greeted by name.

The front desk person looks up, makes eye contact, stands up, and says, **"Hi, Mr. Johnson! It's so good to see you. We'll get you back as soon as possible. Can I get you anything to drink?"**

They walk around the desk. They offer water, coffee from the coffee bar, tea. They make the patient feel seen and welcomed. This takes ten seconds. But it completely changes the patient's experience.

Why it matters for burnout prevention: When your front desk greets patients warmly, patients are already in a good mood when they get to you. They are not tense, defensive, or annoyed. And that makes your job easier.

Now, let's talk about the waiting room itself. Most dental offices smell like a dental office. Antiseptic. Sterile. Clinical. And that smell triggers anxiety. Because people associate it with pain and fear.

Dr. Kalli's parents figured this out in the 1990s. They installed a massive, expensive coffee machine in the waiting room. Not just for convenience. But so the office would smell like coffee instead of formocresol and disinfectant. It worked. Patients walked in and smelled coffee. And they relaxed.

You do not need a $10,000 coffee machine. You can use essential oil diffusers. You can have fresh flowers. You can bake cookies in a small oven in the break room.

The point is: **Pay attention to the sensory experience.**

What does your office smell like? What does it sound like? What does it look like? Because patients are making judgments before they ever sit in your chair. And if the waiting room feels cold, sterile, and unwelcoming, they are already on edge.

But if it feels warm, comfortable, and pleasant, they are relaxed. And relaxed patients are easier to work with.

Retrieving From the Lobby, Not Shouting From the Door

Here is a pet peeve of Dr. Kalli's and it should be yours too.

Most dental offices retrieve patients by shouting their name from a doorway.

"Sharon! Sharon Grossman!"

And the patient, wherever they are in the waiting room, has to gather their things, stand up, and walk toward the voice. It is impersonal. It is lazy. And it feels like being called like cattle. Dr. Kalli's practice does not do that.

Instead, the hygienist, dental assistant, or treatment coordinator **walks all the way out to the waiting room. They go directly to the patient. They greet them by name.**

"Hi, Sharon! I'm so glad you're here. Let's get you back."

And they walk with the patient to the operatory.

Why it matters: This is another touchpoint where you are demonstrating care and attention. The patient feels valued. They feel like you actually care that they are there.

And again, when patients feel cared for, they are easier to work with. They trust you more. They are more likely to accept treatment. They are less likely to complain.

Why it matters for burnout prevention: When your team creates a positive experience from the start, you do not have to work as hard to build rapport. The patient is already on your side.

Dr. Kalli trained her team on this by literally practicing it. She had team members sit in the waiting room, and she made other team members practice walking out, greeting them, and walking them back.

It felt silly at first. But it made a difference. Because if you do not practice it, it feels awkward. And when it feels awkward, people default to shouting from the doorway. If you don't set the expectations to your team that your patients will be retrieved a certain way, it will not happen.

Retrieve from the lobby. Every single time.

The Operatory Setup: Name on Screen, Rear Delivery Protocol

The patient walks into the operatory. What do they see?

In Dr. Kalli's practice, they see their name on the screen.

She uses a simple PowerPoint slide that says: **"This suite has been prepared for you, [Patient Name]."**

It is a small thing. But it is memorable. Patients notice. They feel like you were expecting them. Like you prepared for them specifically.

Why it matters for burnout prevention: When you create small moments of delight for patients, they are less likely to focus on the parts of the experience that are uncomfortable (the needle, the drill, the bill). They are more likely to leave happy. And happy patients do not leave bad reviews.

Now, let's talk about the physical setup.

Dr. Kalli's practice uses rear delivery units. That means the patient is not facing you when you walk in. They are facing a window or a wall.

This creates a challenge: it is easy to stand behind the patient and talk to the back of their head. Talking to the back of someone's head implies they are not important enough for you to make eye contact with.

So Dr. Kalli trained her team (and herself): **Always walk all the way around. Always position yourself in front of the patient, even if it takes an extra five seconds.**

Make eye contact. Let them see your face. Talk to them like a human being, not a head in a chair.

Why it matters for burnout prevention: When you connect with patients face-to-face, you build trust faster. They see you as a person, not just a provider. And that makes difficult conversations (like treatment costs or complex cases) easier.

Also, make sure the operatory is clean. Not just clinically clean, but visually clean.

Dr. Kalli is very clear with her team: "Nothing rages me faster than something on the floor that should have been swept up for the next patient."

If there is debris on the floor, if the tray is not set up, if something looks messy, it reflects poorly on you. And it makes patients question whether you are detail-oriented enough to do good work.

Clean operatory = trust. Messy operatory = doubt.

The Intake That Downloads You Properly

Here is where many practices fail.

The patient is in the chair. The assistant or hygienist talks to them for 15 minutes, gathering information, taking vitals, asking about medical history, figuring out why they are there. And then the dentist walks in and has no idea what just happened. So the patient has to repeat everything. And the dentist looks unprepared.

Dr. Kalli does not tolerate this in her practice.

Her assistants and hygienists are trained to do a thorough intake. And they are trained to **"download" the dentist before the dentist enters the room.**

This can happen in the hallway as the dentist is walking to the operatory. It can happen via a quick text or message. But it happens.

The assistant says: "This is Mrs. Stevenson. She's here because she's been having sensitivity on the lower left. She's nervous about needles. Her blood pressure is 130/80. She mentioned she's interested in Invisalign but wants to focus on the sensitivity first."

Boom. Now the dentist walks in informed. Prepared. Ready to address the patient's concerns without having to ask a hundred questions.

Why it matters for burnout prevention: When you walk into an operatory already knowing what is going on, you save mental energy. You do not have to rebuild context every single time. You can focus on the patient and the problem instead of playing catch-up.

Dr. Kalli is very clear about this: "I don't want to blow into an op and not know what's going on. That makes me look bad."

Train your team to download you. And if they are not doing it, stop before you go into the room and ask, "What do I need to know?"

Do not walk in blind.

Co-Diagnosing: Training Your Team to Sell the Case Before You Enter

Here is where Dr. Kalli's system gets really powerful.

Most dentists think they have to do all the educating, all the case presentation, all the selling. But that is exhausting. And inefficient.

Dr. Kalli trains her hygienists and assistants to **co-diagnose.**

What does that mean?

It means they know what to look for. They know the signs and symptoms of the conditions Dr. Kalli treats most often (like airway issues, for example). And they know how to start the conversation with the patient before Dr. Kalli ever enters the room.

For example, a patient comes in for a cleaning. The hygienist notices that the patient snores, has a small airway, and has wear patterns on their teeth consistent with grinding.

Instead of waiting for Dr. Kalli to point all of this out, the hygienist says:

"Have you ever talked to Dr. Kalli about your airway? I'm noticing a few things that make me think you might benefit from some of the treatments she offers. Have you ever had a sleep study? I'm going to have her come take a look."

Now, when Dr. Kalli walks in, the patient is already primed. They are already thinking about it. The hygienist has planted the seed.

And Dr. Kalli can build on that instead of starting from scratch.

Her hygienists will literally tell patients, "You watch—this is what Dr. Kalli is going to say. She's going to recommend this, this, and this. And I can't wait for her to come in and validate what we've been talking about."

By the time Dr. Kalli arrives, the patient is already halfway to saying yes.

Why it matters for burnout prevention: When your team does the groundwork, you do not have to spend 45 minutes explaining every case. You can confirm what the team has already said, add your expertise, and move forward. This saves you time and mental energy.

But here is the key: **Your team cannot co-diagnose if you have not trained them.**

You have to teach them what to look for. You have to give them scripts. You have to role-play with them so they feel confident.

Dr. Kalli does regular team training. She brings the whole team together and goes over cases, explains her thought process, teaches them the signs and symptoms to watch for. And that investment pays off every single day.

Train your team to co-diagnose. It will change your practice.

The Doctor Experience: Body Language, Confidence, Case Acceptance

Now the dentist enters the room. And everything about how you enter matters.

Dr. Kalli is very intentional about this. She does not rush in, frazzled and distracted. She does not stand behind the patient talking to the back of their head.

She walks in calmly. She positions herself in front of the patient. She makes eye contact. She often puts a hand on the patient's shoulder or forearm to create connection.

Body language matters.

If you are tense, the patient will be tense. If you are calm, the patient will relax.

Dr. Kalli pays attention to her posture, her tone of voice, her facial expression. She consciously slows down her speech if the patient is anxious. She takes deep breaths to regulate her own nervous system. And she diagnoses what she sees.

This sounds obvious, but Dr. Kalli has noticed that many dentists are afraid to tell patients what they see. They are afraid to "spend the patient's money." They are afraid of being seen as pushy or salesy.

So they downplay things. "Well, we could watch this cavity." "You might want to consider orthodontics at some point." This is a mistake.

Dr. Kalli's parents taught her: **"Don't be afraid to spend your patients' money. Tell them what they need and let them make the decision."**

Your job is to diagnose what you see and explain the consequences of treating it versus not treating it. If there is a cavity, say so. If there is bone loss, say so. If there is an airway issue, say so.

And then explain: "Here is what I recommend. Here is why. Here is what happens if we do this. Here is what happens if we don't."

Speak with confidence.

Do not hedge. Do not waffle. Do not say, "I think maybe, possibly, you might need..."

Say, "You need a crown. Here is why."

Patients want clarity. They want confidence. They want to trust that you know what you are doing. And when you speak with confidence, your case acceptance goes up.

Dr. Kalli has a 97% case acceptance rate on airway cases. That is not because she is pushy. It is because she is clear, confident, and thorough in her case presentations.

Why it matters for burnout prevention: When you have high case acceptance, you do not have to work as hard to hit your production goals. You can see fewer patients and still produce more. And that creates space in your schedule. Which reduces burnout.

Also, when patients say yes to treatment, you get to actually help them. And that is fulfilling. That is why you became a dentist.

But when patients keep saying no, it is demoralizing. You start to feel like you are not making a difference.

So speak with confidence. Diagnose what you see. Present treatment clearly. And let the patient decide.

The Laminated Handoff Sheet That Saves Your Sanity

Here is where the system gets really tactical.

When the patient is done in the operatory, they need to get to the front desk to schedule their next appointment and handle payment.

And this is where poor hand off and poor communication wastes time and increases your treatment coordinators stress.

The assistant walks the patient to the front. The front desk says, "How was everything?"

And the assistant says, "Uh, I think Dr. Kalli said they need to come back for a filling?"

The front desk has no idea what procedure, how much time to block, when it needs to be done.

So they check the patient chart. Nothing charted yet. The RDA has already walked away. Now the front desk has to go find the assistant or the dentist to ask. All while the patient is standing there ready to go home, with a numb face and an experience that probably hurt!

It is chaotic. It is inefficient. And things fall through the cracks.

Dr. Kalli solved this with a **laminated handoff sheet.**

The assistant fills it out before leaving the operatory. It includes:

- Patient name
- Procedure that was done (if any)
- Procedure that needs to be scheduled
- How much time to block for the next appointment (critical!)
- Timeline ("Dr. Kalli wants this done within two weeks")
- Any special notes

Then the assistant walks the patient to the front desk and **does a verbal handoff in front of the patient.**

"Hi, I've got Mr. Smith here. We had a great experience today. He's going to need a few fillings done, Dr. Kalli wants to start on the upper right and she wants this done within the next two weeks. She needs no less than 90 minutes for the appointment."

Now the front desk has everything they need. And the patient has heard it, so there is no confusion later. The patient hearing it more than one time is so important!

Why it matters for burnout prevention: When handoffs are clean, nothing falls through the cracks. Patients actually schedule. Your treatment acceptance rate will increase dramatically.The front desk does not interrupt you in the middle of another appointment to ask questions. Everything flows.

Dr. Kalli is strict about this. Her treatment coordinators know, if the assistant tries to hand off a patient without filling out the sheet, they are supposed to send them back to fill it out. Because the system only works if everyone follows it.

Create a handoff protocol. Make it non-negotiable. Remember, you get what you tolerate.

Exit Experience: Post-Op Calls, Review Requests, Follow-Up Cadence

The patient leaves. The appointment is over.

But the experience is not.

Dr. Kalli's practice does **post-op calls** for every patient who had a shot, any kind of invasive procedure, or expressed anxiety. *Anyone who experienced discomfort.*

Morning patients are called at lunch. Afternoon patients are called the next morning.

The call is simple:

"Hi, Mrs. Wilson! This is Sarah calling from Dr. Kalli's office. We just wanted to check in and see how you're feeling after your appointment today. Any pain or concerns?"

Most patients say, "Oh, I'm fine! Thanks so much for calling."

And that is it. A 30-second call.

But the impact is huge. Because most dental offices do not do this. So when you do, patients are shocked. And delighted.

They tell their friends, "My dentist actually called to check on me!"

Why it matters for burnout prevention: Happy patients leave good reviews. They refer their friends. They do not complain or leave negative feedback. And that reduces your stress.

Speaking of reviews: **Dr. Kalli's practice asks for reviews at multiple touchpoints.**

The assistant asks in the operatory while the patient is still numb: "Would you mind leaving us a Google review? Here's a QR code—you can scan it right now."

The front desk asks at checkout: "Did you have a great experience today? We'd love it if you'd leave us a review."

They have QR codes everywhere—on the checkout desk, in every operatory, on business cards. And they make it easy. Scan the code, leave the review. Done.

Why this matters: You need good reviews to counterbalance the inevitable bad reviews. And you will not get reviews if you do not ask.

Finally, there is a **follow-up cadence for unscheduled treatment.**

If a patient says no to a treatment plan, they do not just disappear. They get a call two weeks later.

"Hi, Mr. Blake. Dr. Kalli has been thinking about you. She's really concerned about that tooth we talked about. We'd love to get you in before it gets worse. Would a morning or afternoon appointment work best?" *Avoid yes or no questions.*

You are not begging. You are not being pushy. You are being genuinely concerned. And many patients say yes when they are called. Because the initial no was often about timing or fear, not about not wanting the treatment.

Why it matters for burnout prevention: Unscheduled treatment is lost revenue. And lost revenue means you have to see more patients to hit your goals. But when you follow up, you convert more cases. And that means you can see fewer patients overall. *If you never follow up, how will you know the real reason they didn't schedule?*

Reflection Questions:

1. Which part of your patient experience is most chaotic right now? Where are you improvising instead of following a system?
2. What is one script or protocol you could create this week that would reduce stress for you and your team?

3. How are you currently training your team to co-diagnose and prepare patients before you enter the room? What could improve?
4. When was the last time you audited your phone calls, patient flow, or handoffs? What might you discover if you listened or observed?
5. If you created a visual map of your patient experience, where would the breakdowns be? What would you fix first?

CHAPTER 8

Build Your A-Team Without Burning Yourself Out

Dr. Kalli Hale will never forget the Thursday afternoon when Katherine quit.

She was at piano lessons with her kids. Her phone rang. Dr. Kyle's voice on the other end: "Katherine just quit."

For a moment, Dr. Kalli could not process it. Katherine. Her lead assistant. The person she had invested in, trained, taken to conferences, trusted implicitly. The person she thought was loyal.

Gone.

And not just gone—gone abruptly, without warning, leaving Dr. Kalli to figure out how to cover a full schedule without her right-hand person.

Dr. Kalli felt deep anger. Betrayed. Like she had given everything to Katherine and gotten nothing in return. But looking back, she can see it differently now.

The problem was not that Katherine quit. The problem was that Dr. Kalli had created a dynamic where one person quitting could feel like the end of the world. She had gotten too close. She had made Katherine indispensable. She had ignored warning signs of dysfunction because she was afraid of losing Katherine. And when Katherine finally left, it exposed every weakness in how Dr. Kalli was leading her team.

That experience taught her something critical: **You cannot build a sustainable practice on the backs of individuals. You have to build it on systems.**

Your team should be excellent. But no single person should be irreplaceable. Including you.

Your relationships with staff should be warm. But they cannot be so personal that you lose objectivity.

You should invest in your people. But you also need to protect yourself from being held hostage by them.

This is the balance that most practice owners struggle with. And it is the balance that, when you get it right, transforms your practice from chaotic and dependent to smooth and sustainable.

This chapter is about building an A-team without burning yourself out in the process.

The User Manual You Need to Create (And What Goes In It)

Here is a question: If you got hit by a bus tomorrow, could someone else run your practice? For most dentists, the answer is no. Because everything is in your head. The protocols you follow. The decisions you make. The way you like things done. Your team knows bits and pieces. But no one has the whole picture. And that is a problem. Not just for business continuity. But for your daily stress level.

Because if everything depends on you—if you are the only one who knows how things should be done—then you can never step back. You can never delegate fully. You are always the bottleneck.

Dr. Kalli learned this the hard way. And she fixed it by creating what she calls **the practice user manual.**

It is a comprehensive document (now digital, but it started as a binder) that contains:

1. Your practice philosophy and values.

What do you stand for? What kind of care do you provide? What is your mission?

This is not fluff. This is the foundation that guides every decision your team makes when you are not there.

Dr. Kalli's practice values health-conscious, preventive care with a focus on airway and whole-body wellness. That is in the manual. So when a new patient calls asking for the cheapest, fastest fix, the front desk knows: this is probably not the right fit.

2. Phone protocols.

Exactly how to answer the phone. Word-for-word scripts for common questions. How to handle insurance inquiries. How to schedule different types of appointments.

3. Patient flow procedures.

How patients should be greeted. How they should be walked back. How rooms should be set up. What happens if a patient is late. What happens if the schedule is running behind.

4. Clinical protocols.

Which procedures require which setups. Which materials you prefer for which situations. How long to block for different procedures. What your preferences are (music, lighting, assistant positioning, etc.).

5. Emergency procedures.

What to do if a patient has a medical emergency. Who to call. What equipment to grab. Who is responsible for what.

6. Financial policies.

How to discuss costs with patients. What payment options you offer. How to handle financing. What to do if a patient cannot pay.

7. Team roles and responsibilities.

Who is responsible for what. Who backs up whom. What decisions can be made without asking you.

8. Training expectations.

How new employees are onboarded. What they need to learn in the first week, first month, first three months. Who trains them on what.

Why this matters for burnout prevention:

When you have a user manual, you do not have to answer the same questions over and over. Your team can reference the manual. They can train new employees using the manual. They can make decisions confidently because they know what you expect. And that takes the mental load off you.

Dr. Kalli is very clear about this: "Hosting training for your teams is probably the most important thing you are forgetting to do in your practice. It needs to be ongoing."

But training is exhausting if you have to do it from scratch every time. The manual makes it repeatable. Scalable. Sustainable.

Start creating your user manual today. You do not have to do it all at once. Start with one section. Write down the protocol for how you want the phone answered. Then move to the next thing.

Over time, you build a comprehensive guide that makes your practice run smoothly whether you are there or not. And that is freedom.

Earning Respect Without Being Scary (Or Their Best Friend)

Dr. Kalli struggled with this in the early years of her career.

In the beginning, staff members told the office manager they were afraid of her. She was not yelling? She was not throwing instruments? This news actually shocked her. But her intensity—her perfectionism, her frustration with herself when things did not go perfectly—created an atmosphere of tension. She also held her teams to high expectations that some were not used to prior to working for her. *You get what you tolerate.*

Later, she swung the other way. She became too close with Katherine. And that closeness created blind spots. She ignored dysfunction. She tolerated behavior from Katherine that she would not have tolerated from anyone else.

Why? Because she didn't know how her practice would survive without Katherine's help. Neither extreme worked.

So what is the right balance?

Here is what Dr. Kalli has learned: **You earn respect by being consistent, fair, and clear.** Not by being their boss in a way that makes them fear you. Not by being their friend in a way that makes you lose authority. But by being a leader who has high standards and also genuinely cares about their wellbeing.

What this looks like in practice:

1. Be warm, but maintain professional distance.

Greet your team every morning. Ask how they are doing. Show interest in their lives. Celebrate their wins.

But do not make one person your confidant. Do not share things with one employee that you would not share with the whole team. Do not create special relationships that breed favoritism.

2. Set clear expectations and hold people accountable.

Your team should know exactly what is expected of them. And if they do not meet those expectations, there should be consequences. Not punishment. But accountability. A conversation. A plan to improve. And if improvement does not happen, a decision about whether this is the right fit.

Dr. Kalli is very clear: "You have to earn their respect. You need to talk to them. But they also need to know that you're the boss. They need to know that you expect them to get their job done so that your patients are served well."

3. Do not avoid difficult conversations.

This is where most practice owners fail. They see a problem—an employee who is not performing, a dynamic that is not working—and they avoid addressing it because they do not want conflict.

But avoidance does not make the problem go away. It makes it fester.

Dr. Kalli's father gave her advice early on: If an employee complains about you to someone else instead of talking to you directly, you need to address it. Immediately.

She remembers the time an assistant was upset about something Dr. Kalli said and went to her dad to complain. He came to Dr. Kalli and said, "You need to talk to her."

Dr. Kalli did not want to. It was uncomfortable. But she did it. And the conversation cleared the air. *These conversations always go worse in your mind - deep breaths and clarity on what needs to be said without emotions being involved is important.*

If you avoid difficult conversations, you lose respect. Because your team sees that you will not address problems. And that creates resentment and dysfunction. They also see what they can get away with, because, again: *you get what you tolerate.*

4. Acknowledge when you are wrong.

You are not perfect. You will make mistakes. You will have bad days. You will say things you should not say.

When that happens, own it. Apologize. Make it right.

Dr. Kalli describes a time when she was so stressed that her demeanor in the operatory was tense and sharp. Her team felt it. She could have been defensive. But instead, she acknowledged it. "Please don't take my attitude personally. You are doing a great job and my stress level is affecting how I communicate. I apologize for that!"

That vulnerability actually builds respect. Because your team sees that you are human. That you are willing to grow. That you care about how you affect them.

The balance is this: Care about your team without making them your emotional support system. Lead with clarity without leading with fear.

Daily Deposits: Checking In Without Hovering

One of the simplest but most powerful leadership practices Dr. Kalli learned is this:

Check in with your team every morning.

Not in a micromanaging way. Not in a "what have you done for me lately" way. But in a genuine, human way. Walk around the office before the first patient. Say good morning to everyone. Look them in the eye. Ask, "Is there anything I can do for you today? Anything you need from me?"

It takes five minutes. Maybe less. But it sets the tone for the day. Your team knows you see them. You care. You are available if they need you.

And when problems arise during the day, they feel comfortable bringing them to you because you have already established that you are approachable.

We call this making daily deposits.

You are depositing goodwill, connection, and trust. So that when you need to make a withdrawal—when you need to give critical feedback or ask someone to stay late or handle a difficult situation—you have equity in the relationship.

But here is the key: **Check in without hovering.**

You are not standing over their shoulder watching everything they do. You are not questioning every decision. You are not inserting yourself into every situation. You are making yourself available. And then you are stepping back and letting them do their jobs.

This is especially important for dentists who struggle with control issues (*which, let's be honest, is most dentists*). You have to trust your team to do their jobs. And if you cannot trust them, you either need to train them better or hire different people. *Always keep your "bench" full [hiring]. Keeping someone in the wrong seat for too long is a mistake every dentist makes at least once.*

But you cannot build a sustainable practice if you are micromanaging every detail.

The daily check-in is enough. It keeps you connected without keeping you enmeshed.

Training as Ongoing Practice, Not One-Time Event

Most dental practices do training once: when an employee is hired. They show them the ropes. They explain the basics. And then they assume the employee knows what to do forever. This is a mistake.

Training is not a one-time event. It is an ongoing practice. *How do you communicate changes to procedures with your team, if you only train once?*

Dr. Kalli does regular team training. Sometimes it is clinical—going over new procedures, explaining her approach to certain cases, teaching them what to look for.

Sometimes it is operational—reviewing the phone scripts, walking through the patient flow, auditing the handoff process.

Sometimes it is just team-building—getting everyone together to talk about what is working and what is not. But it is consistent. It is scheduled. It is non-negotiable.

Why this matters for burnout prevention:

When your team is well-trained, they do not come to you with every question. They know what to do. They feel confident. And that reduces the mental load on you.

But when your team is under-trained, you are constantly putting out fires. Answering questions. Fixing mistakes. Cleaning up after them. *Exacerbating your decision fatigue.*

And that is exhausting.

Dr. Kalli describes doing a whole lecture for her team on airway management. She brought everyone together—front desk, hygienists, assistants—and walked them through what she does, why she does it, and what they should be looking for.

And now, her hygienists can start the airway conversation with patients before she even enters the room. Her front desk can explain airway treatments when patients call with questions. Her assistants know how to set up for airway procedures without asking. *What dentist wouldn't appreciate a few less questions to answer?*

That is the power of training.

Schedule regular training sessions. Quarterly at minimum for bigger topics that require more than one hour. Monthly for one hour, if you can.

And make attendance mandatory. Because if training is optional, it sends the message that it is not important. *Yes, you pay your teams when you ask them to come to training. If it's during their lunch break, you provide lunch also.*

Your team's competence is directly tied to your stress level. Invest in it.

The Power of Awareness Tools

We've touched on many of these strategies throughout the book, but they all fall under one powerful umbrella: the concept of **Awareness Tools**.

An Awareness Tool is a small, physical reminder designed to keep your team conscious of a specific desired behavior. Instead of asking your team to exert more mental energy, these tools use environmental cues to make the "right way" the easiest way. When you shift the burden from a person's memory to a physical tool, you create a system that supports the human.

Here are some awareness tools Dr. Kalli has used:

- **Front Desk Mirrors:** Dr. Kalli placed a mirror by the phone so that every time a team member reached for the receiver, they saw their reflection. It served as a visual cue to smile, ensuring a warm and professional tone with every patient.
- **Laminated Handoff Sheets:** To ensure clean transitions from the operatory to the front desk, use a physical form. Making the handoff visual and tactile makes it a concrete part of the process.
- **Strategic QR Codes:** If you want more patient reviews, place QR codes in the operatories and at checkout. The easier the tool makes the task, the more likely it is to happen.
- **Visual Setup Guides:** Post checklists and laminated photos of tray setups in every room. This allows new employees to reference them instantly and experienced staff to double-check their work.

- **Stationary Phone Scripts:** Post scripts where the front desk can see them at eye level. They don't have to memorize every word; they can simply glance at the script to stay on track.

Why this matters for burnout prevention:

When you rely on people to remember everything, things fall through the cracks. And then you have to fix it. Or remind them. Or redo it yourself. But when you create visual reminders and tools, people do not have to rely on memory. The system supports them. And that reduces errors. Which reduces stress. Which prevents burnout.

Think about the behaviors you want from your team. Then create tools that make those behaviors easier.

Recording Calls and Auditing Your Team's Patient Interactions

Dr. Kalli uses a phone system that records every call.

And she listened to them for years. Until she trusted her office manager to take over that job.If you don't listen to your employees on the phone, how will you know if they're treating patients the way you want them to be treated? Listening to the calls can also help identify where patients are being lost. Where the scripts are not being followed. Where the team needs more training.

If you don't know how they're answering questions on the phone, you cannot verify if they built value for the practice. You also won't know where you need to focus your training for these employees.

And those small failures compound into lost patients. Which means holes in the schedule. Which means lower production. Which means more pressure to see more patients to make up the difference.

Recording and auditing is not optional if you want a high-performing practice.

You cannot fix what you cannot see. And you cannot see what is happening on phone calls unless you listen.

Dr. Kalli also does this with case presentations. She records herself (with patient permission) doing consultations. And then she watches them later. She uses these now to train dentists on how they can improve their patient interactions.

At first, it was uncomfortable. She noticed how many times she said "um." She noticed moments where she was not as clear as she could have been. She noticed body language that did not convey confidence. But watching herself allowed her to improve. And now her case acceptance is over 97%.

If you are not recording and auditing, you are flying blind.

Set up a system to record calls. Set aside time monthly to listen to a sample. Identify patterns. Retrain where needed. This is not about being controlling. This is about creating excellence.

What Are You Tolerating? The Question That Changes Everything

Here is a powerful question Dr. Kalli asks practice owners:

What are you tolerating?

What behavior from your team are you putting up with that you know is not okay?

What dysfunction are you ignoring because you do not want to deal with it?

What mediocrity are you accepting because you are afraid of losing someone?

For Dr. Kalli, she was tolerating Katherine's treatment of the rest of the staff. She was tolerating the discord Katherine was creating because she was afraid of losing her.

And that tolerance cost her. It cost her team morale. It cost her respect. And eventually, it cost her Katherine anyway.

Most practice owners are tolerating something. Maybe it is:

- An employee who is consistently late

- A team member who does the bare minimum (who is picking up their slack?)
- Someone who gossips or creates drama
- A front desk person who is rude to patients
- An assistant who does not follow protocols
- A hygienist who does not co-diagnose with you

Whatever it is, it is costing you in time, in money, and worse, in morale. Because what you tolerate becomes the standard.

If you tolerate lateness, why would they show up on time for you?.

If you tolerate mediocrity, why should they go above and beyond for your patients?.

If you tolerate disrespect, you will lose the respect of the rest of the team.

Your tolerance is your team's permission.

So ask yourself: What am I tolerating? And why?

Usually, the answer is fear. Fear of confrontation. Fear of losing the person. Fear that you will not find someone better.

But here is the truth: **The cost of tolerating dysfunction is higher than the cost of addressing it.**

Even if addressing it means someone leaves.

Even if it means you have to hire and train someone new.

Even if it means a difficult conversation.

Stop tolerating. Start leading.

Delegation Without Losing Control

Dentists struggle with delegation. You want everything done perfectly. You assume no one else can do it as well as you. So you do it yourself.And then you burn out because you are carrying everything.

Dr. Kalli had to learn to delegate. And it was not easy.

She had to tolerate the discomfort of things not being done exactly the way she would do them. She had to accept that mistakes would happen. She had to trust that her team could learn.

But here is what she discovered: Delegation does not mean losing control. It means creating systems that allow others to execute to your standards.

So how do you delegate effectively?

1. Identify tasks that do not require your clinical expertise.

Calling the lab to check on a case. Ordering supplies. Scheduling follow-ups. Pulling charts. Confirming appointments.

None of these require you. But if you are doing them, you are wasting time you could spend doing clinical work or business strategy.

2. Train the person thoroughly.

Do not just say, "Call the lab." Show them what to ask. Give them a script. Walk them through it the first time. Then let them do it while you observe. Then let them do it on their own.

3. Create accountability systems.

If you delegate scheduling follow-ups, create a system to track it. A list. A report. Something that shows you it is getting done.

You are not micromanaging. You are creating visibility.

4. Let go of perfection.

The task might not be done exactly the way you would do it. And that is okay. As long as it is done to an acceptable standard, let it go.

Dr. Kalli talks about this: "Delegation is about empowering other people to meet high standards so you don't have to carry everything alone." Don't fix your employees' mistakes, help them fix them! If you ask your employee to write a protocol for room turnover, don't edit it afterwards yourself. Tell them the changes you want made and empower them to edit it for your review again later.

The goal is not to do everything yourself. The goal is to build a team that can do everything without you.

When to Fire Someone (And Why You Should Never Rehire Them)

This is the part dentists don't want to do. But sometimes, you have to fire someone.

And if you have never done it, it feels impossible. You agonize over it. You delay. You hope the problem will fix itself.

But it does not.

Here is when you need to fire someone:

1. They are not doing the job despite training and feedback.

You have trained them. You have given clear expectations. You have had conversations about what needs to improve. And nothing changes.

At that point, it is not about them being a bad person. It is about this not being the right fit.

2. They are creating toxicity in the team.

Gossip. Drama. Undermining. Disrespect. These are not tolerable.

Even if the person is clinically skilled, if they are poisoning the culture, they have to go.

3. They are dishonest or unethical.

This is non-negotiable. Lying, stealing, cutting corners, violating patient trust—any of these is an immediate termination.

How to do it:

Do not drag it out. Do not give endless chances. If you have decided, do it quickly and cleanly.

Have the conversation in private. Be direct. "I know this is hard to hear, but it's not a decision I am willing to change."

Do not over-explain. Do not get into a debate. Repeat the above, over and over, no dramatic details about why you are firing them. Just state the decision and move on.

And here is the critical part: **Never rehire them. When someone is gone, they stay gone.**

Handling Staff Conflicts Before They Explode

Most staff conflicts do not start as explosions. They start as small tensions that you ignore.

Two people who do not communicate well. A passive-aggressive comment. A feeling of unfairness about workload or schedule.

And you think, *It's fine. They'll work it out.*

But they do not work it out. It festers. It spreads. It becomes a bigger problem.

Dr. Kalli learned this with Katherine. The dysfunction between Katherine and the rest of the staff did not happen overnight. It was built over months. Maybe years.

And Dr. Kalli had no idea it was going on. It was being hidden from her to an extent, but also she didn't check on the team. Truth be told, she did not want to deal with it.

But ignoring it did not make it go away. It just made it worse.

How to handle conflicts:

1. Address them early.

If you sense tension, say something. Pull the people aside individually. Ask what is going on. Listen.

Do not wait for it to blow up.

2. Do not take sides.

Your job is not to decide who is right. Your job is to create an environment where people can work together professionally.

So listen to both sides. Acknowledge both perspectives. And then set clear expectations: "Here is how I need you two to work together moving forward."

3. Make it about behavior, not personality.

Do not say, "You're being difficult." Say, "When you speak to her that way, it creates tension. I need you to communicate more respectfully."

Focus on the specific behavior you want to change.

4. If it cannot be resolved, make a decision.

Sometimes, people just do not work well together. And if mediation does not fix it, you have to decide: Who stays, and who goes?

This is hard. But it is your job as a leader.

Unresolved conflict is one of the biggest drains on practice morale and your own energy. Handle it before it explodes.

The Katherine Lesson: Professional Boundaries That Protect You

Let's come back to Katherine. Because the Katherine story is not just about one employee quitting. It is about the danger of tolerating poor behavior from a team member.

Dr. Kalli made Katherine special. She invested in her. She took her to trainings. She trusted her with everything. And that closeness created blind spots.

Here is the lesson: You can care about your team without making them your inner circle.

You can invest in them. Train them. Support them. Celebrate them. But you cannot make one person indispensable. You cannot get so close that you lose objectivity. Because when you do, you create a power dynamic that is unhealthy for everyone.

Katherine knew she was special. She used it. She treated other staff members poorly because she knew Dr. Kalli would not hold her accountable. And the rest of the team resented it.

Professional boundaries protect everyone.

They protect you from being manipulated or held hostage.

They protect the team from favoritism and dysfunction.

They protect the employee from having inappropriate expectations placed on them.

Build a team. Not a family. Not an inner circle.

Where everyone is valued. Where everyone is held to the same standards. Where no one is irreplaceable. That is how you build something sustainable.

What This All Means

Building an A-team is not about finding perfect people.

It is about creating systems, setting clear expectations, providing ongoing training, and maintaining healthy boundaries.

It is about leading with clarity and compassion.

It is about addressing problems early instead of letting them fester.

It is about delegating without losing control.

It is about making daily deposits so you have equity when you need to make withdrawals.

And most importantly, it is about recognizing that ***your team's competence and morale directly affect your stress level.***

If your team is well-trained, empowered, and aligned with your vision, your practice runs smoothly. And you can focus on the work that only you can do. Dr. Kalli's parents often said: *the dentistry is the easy part.*

If your team is dysfunctional, undertrained, or dependent on you for every decision, you will burn out trying to hold it all together.

Invest in your team. Build systems. Set boundaries. Lead well.

And you will build a practice that does not drain you—it energizes you.

Because you are not doing it alone. You have a team that supports you, executes to your standards, and makes your vision a reality.

That is how you build something that lasts.

Reflection Questions:

1. Do you have a user manual for your practice? If not, what is one section you could start writing this week?
2. What are you currently tolerating from your team that you know is not okay? What would it take to address it?
3. Are there tasks you are doing that do not require your clinical expertise? What could you delegate this week?
4. Have you gotten too close to any employee in a way that has created blind spots? What boundaries do you need to set?
5. When was the last time you invested in team training? What is one training session you could schedule in the next 30 days?

CHAPTER 9

Designing A Career That Lasts

Here is a mistake Dr. Kalli made for years: all of her time in the work week was spent seeing patients. Seems counterintuitive, right? You're a dentist. You should see patients all day.

If she was in the operatory, she was productive. If she was not, she wasn't making money. So she packed her clinical schedule. Every hour, every day. Because that was how you made money, right?

But here is what she did not account for: **You are not just a clinician. You are also a business owner.**

And running a business requires time. Time to review financials. Time to train staff. Time to develop systems. Time to plan for growth. If you do not block time for business work during business hours, you end up doing it at night and on weekends. Which means you never stop working.

Dr. Kalli's turning point came when Dr. Kyle forced her to block off Tuesdays. And that shift was revelatory. Now she had time to work on herself. Read leadership books. Recover from burnout. Sit with her thoughts and recover from decision fatigue.

She used Tuesday mornings to read, to learn, to work through *The Burnout Solution.* She used Tuesday afternoons to review the practice's financials, to plan new systems, to think strategically about where she wanted the practice to go. What her personal goals were going to be. What her professional goals were going to be.

And something remarkable happened: **The practice thrived because the leader she was meant to be finally shined.**

Because she was finally working *on* the business instead of just *in* it.

She identified bottlenecks in the schedule. She redesigned the patient flow. She created training protocols. She hired strategically.

Here is the principle: Time spent working on your business is not wasted. It is an investment that multiplies your effectiveness. If you don't work on your business, you will lose your business.

But you have to protect it. You have to block it on your schedule. And you have to treat it as non-negotiable.

Dr. Kalli now blocks time every week for business work. Sometimes it is Monday afternoons. Sometimes it is a full day. But it is always there.

And during that time, she is not in the building.

If you want to build something sustainable, you have to make time to think, plan, and strategize.

Not just react. Not just survive. But actually design. And breathe.

The Schedule Evolution: From Chaos to Intentional Design

Dr. Kalli's schedule has evolved dramatically over the years.

Phase 1: The grind (early career)

Four full days a week, 8 a.m. to 5 p.m., packed with patients. No breaks. No lunch. 140 new patients a month. Seeing everyone who called. In-network with every insurance. Saying yes to everything.

Then: BURNOUT

Phase 2: The first boundary (recovery phase)

Dr. Kyle forced her to cut Tuesdays. She went from four days to three days of clinical work, with Tuesday off the premises for recovery and business work.

The practice did not collapse. In fact, it improved. Because she came back refreshed. And she started building systems that reduced chaos.

Phase 3: Strategic blocking (growth phase)

As she hired associate dentists, she started being more intentional about her clinical time. She stopped seeing every patient. She focused on the cases she loved—complex airway cases, patients who valued her expertise, cases that challenged her clinically.

She blocked Monday afternoons for business work. She stopped working past 3 p.m. on Fridays so she could pick her kids up from school.

Phase 4: Leverage and leadership (current phase)

Now, Dr. Kalli works clinically maybe two to three days a week. The rest of her time is spent on leadership—overseeing the eight practices, mentoring other dentists, building the teledentistry company, speaking at conferences.

Her income is no longer tied to how many hours she spends in the operatory. Because she has built leverage. She has associate dentists producing in multiple locations. She has other income streams.

The lesson: Your schedule should evolve as your career evolves.

What works in your first five years will not work in your next ten. And what works when you are single and childless will not work when you have a family.

You have to be intentional about redesigning your schedule to match the phase of life and career you are in.

Ask yourself:

- What do I want my week to look like right now?
- What kind of cases do I want to spend my time on?
- How much time do I need for business work versus clinical work?
- What boundaries do I need to protect my family time?

And then design your schedule accordingly.

Do not just accept the default. Do not just keep doing what you have always done because that is how it has always been. *"If you always do what you've always done, you'll always get what you've always got." - Jessie Potter (Dr. Kalli's dad)*

Design on purpose.

Work-Life Integration for Dentists With Families

The phrase "work-life balance" is misleading.

It implies that work and life are two separate things that need to be equally weighted. Like you spend eight hours at work, eight hours with your family, eight hours sleeping, and everything is balanced.

But that is not reality. Especially for practice owners. Work and life are not separate. They are integrated. They bleed into each other.

So the question is not "How do I balance work and life?" The question is "How do I integrate work and life in a way that honors what matters most to me?"

For Dr. Kalli, what mattered most was being present for her kids. She did not want a nanny raising them forever while she worked 50 hours a week. She did not want to miss school events, pickups, and bedtime. But she also loved dentistry. She loved helping patients. She loved building something. So she had to figure out: **How do I do both?**

The answer was not working less and making less money. The answer was **working differently.**

She hired associate dentists so the practice could produce revenue even when she was not there.

She blocked her clinical schedule so she only worked when her kids were in school.

She built systems so the practice ran smoothly without her needing to be involved in every decision.

She created multiple income streams so she was not dependent on clinical production alone.

And she was ruthless about protecting her boundaries.

When her kids got out of school at 3 p.m., she was done for the day. No exceptions. No "just one more patient." No staying late because the schedule was running behind. *The luxury of being a dentist includes not having to be "on call". Very few "life or death" situations occur in general dentistry.*

If the schedule was running behind, that was a systems problem to fix—not a reason to sacrifice time with her kids.

Here is what work-life integration looks like:

You do not try to separate work and life into neat boxes. You design them to fit together in a way that serves your values.

For Dr. Kalli, that meant:

- Working clinically while her kids were in school
- Picking them up every day
- Doing business work during nap time Traveling for speaking engagements occasionally, but not excessively
- Building businesses that gave her flexibility and leverage

For you, it might look different. Maybe you do not have kids. Maybe you do, but they are older and do not need you as much. Maybe you are caring for aging parents. Maybe you value travel and want to work part-time.

The point is not to copy someone else's model. The point is to **design your career around your values.** And then build systems that make that design possible.

Picking Up Your Kids vs. Seeing the 4 p.m. Patient

Dr. Kalli remembers the moment she decided: **I am picking my kids up from school. Every day. No exceptions.**

This was stressful for her team. Because it meant turning down revenue. It meant blocking her schedule so she was not available after 3 p.m. It meant saying no to patients who could only come at 4 or 5.

And her team pushed back. "But what if a patient really needs to be seen and can only come at 4?"

Dr. Kalli's answer: "Then they see one of the associate doctors. Or they come at a different time. But I am not available after 3."

This felt radical. Selfish, even.

But here is what Dr. Kalli realized: **You only get one chance to raise your kids.**

Patients will always be there. Cases will always be there. But her kids were only going to be little once. And she did not want to look back in 20 years and realize she missed it because she was too busy seeing the 4 p.m. patient. The patient who would never appreciate that sacrifice anyway? So she made the decision. And she enforced it.

This is the shift that prevents burnout long-term.

You stop sacrificing what matters most for what seems urgent. You stop saying yes to everything and everyone. You start designing your work around your life instead of the other way around. And you accept that this might mean saying no to some opportunities, some patients, some revenue. But what you gain is worth infinitely more: presence, peace, and a life you do not want to escape from.

And guess what? She'd earned that privilege.

Building Multiple Practices Without Multiplying Burnout

When Dr. Kyle first came to Dr. Kalli about opening more practices, she was extremely hesitant.

I can barely manage one practice without losing my mind. How are we going to manage more?

But here is what she learned: **More practices do not mean more work—if you build them with leverage and systems from the start.**

The mistake most dentists make when they open a second (or third, or fourth) location is they try to replicate themselves. They think, *I'll just do what I did in the first practice.* But that does not scale. You cannot be in eight places at once.

So Dr. Kalli and her team built differently.

She hired associate dentists for each location. Strong clinicians who could deliver excellent care without needing her to be there every day.

She created systems—the patient experience framework we discussed in Chapter 7—that could be replicated across all locations. Every practice runs the same way. Same phone scripts. Same patient flow. Same standards.

She hired strong office managers for each location who could handle day-to-day operations without constant input from her.

And she built infrastructure: centralized billing, centralized marketing, centralized training.

So instead of managing eight separate businesses, she is managing one business with eight locations.

Here is the key insight: You scale through systems and people, not through personal effort.

If you try to scale by working harder, you will burn out. But if you scale by building systems and empowering people, you can grow without drowning.

Dr. Kalli's role has shifted from clinician to leader. She is not in the operatory every day at every location. She is overseeing the vision, the culture, the strategy.

And that shift has given her more freedom, not less.

If you want to grow, build for leverage from the beginning. Do not wait until you are overwhelmed to start delegating and systematizing.

Design each new location to run without you. And then your growth becomes sustainable instead of suffocating.

From Clinical Dentistry to Leadership and Legacy

At some point in every dentist's career, a fundamental shift occurs. You realize that while you began as a clinician, you now need to become a leader.

For some, this happens when they hire their first associate; for others, it's the moment they realize their business is struggling. But the core truth is the same: **Your value is no longer just in what you do with your hands. It is in what you build with your mind.**

Dr. Kalli experienced this shift only after reaching a breaking point. Her lack of systems and poor scheduling created a "clinical fog" that prevented her from seeing the bigger picture. She loved the operatory, but she hated what the grind was doing to her mental health and her time.

As she began hiring associates and opening new locations, she discovered the power of **leverage**:

- One excellent dentist can treat perhaps 2,000 patients a year.
- One excellent leader who supports ten dentists can impact 20,000+ lives.

By building systems instead of just filling cavities, Dr. Kalli's teledentistry company has treated over 12,000 children in just two years. That is the difference between a job and a legacy. Dr. Kalli's physical locations grew from two to ten in three years! She could never have accomplished this without systems and the understanding that her reach was bigger if she wasn't stuck to the chair.

The Four Phases of a Sustainable Career

Most dentists view their career as a flat line: you see patients until you retire. But that isn't sustainable physically or mentally. To avoid burnout, you must evolve through these four distinct phases:

- **Phase 1: Learn and Build (Years 1–10)**Focused on clinical excellence and "getting your reps." You are building your patient base and learning the ropes of business. This is the time for hustle, but it is a season, not a permanent state.
- **Phase 2: Systematize and Scale (Years 10–20)** The transition from technician to leader. This is where you implement **Awareness Tools** and systems so the practice can run without your constant physical presence. You begin hiring associates and creating multiple income streams.
- **Phase 3: Lead and Mentor (Years 20–30)** Your role shifts from *doing* to *teaching*. You leverage your wisdom by training other dentists, consulting, or expanding your organizational leadership.

- **Phase 4: Legacy and Transition (Years 30+)** Intentionally designing your exit. You are building something that thrives without you, ensuring your impact on the profession lasts long after you hang up the handpiece.

Thought Leadership: Impact Beyond the Chair

As Dr. Kalli recovered from burnout, she realized her experience was a tool in itself. She began saying "yes" to the speaking circuit—podcasts, conferences, and webinars.

This is the highest form of leverage. When you share what you've learned through trial, error, and recovery, you prevent others from suffering the same way. Every time a peer says, *"I thought I was the only one struggling; you gave me hope,"* your impact expands far beyond the four walls of your operatory.

The Key is to Think Ahead.

Do not wait until you are 55 and exhausted to ask "what's next?" Look at the phase you are in today and ask: *What systems am I building now to support the person I will be in ten years?*

Dr. Kalli's Transformation: From Almost Quitting to 10+ Locations

Let's come back to where this chapter started. Dr. Kalli was burned out. Maxed out. Convinced that the only way out was to walk away from dentistry entirely. But she did not quit. She rebuilt.

She read *The Burnout Solution.* She worked through the exercises. She changed how she thought about her work. She blocked off Tuesdays. She started setting boundaries. She hired help. She built systems. She got out of network with insurance. She created the Patient First by SleepWell framework that reduced chaos. She trained her team. She delegated. She focused on her ideal patients instead of trying to serve everyone. And slowly, the practice transformed.

She went from barely surviving to thriving. From working four packed clinical days to one. From doing everything herself to building a team that could run things without her.

And then she started growing. Not because she needed more revenue. But because she had a model that worked and she wanted to share it.

She opened a second location. Then a third. Then a fourth.

She built a teledentistry company.

She started mentoring other dentists.

She began speaking at conferences.

And now, in 2026, she oversees over 10 practice locations. She runs multiple businesses. She mentors dozens of dentists. She is building a legacy. And she picks her kids up from school every day.

This is what is possible when you stop surviving and start designing.

When you stop believing that burnout is the price of success and start building systems that support sustainability.

When you stop trying to do everything yourself and start building leverage.

When you stop reacting to circumstances and start creating the career you actually want.

Dr. Kalli's transformation was not luck. It was intentional design.

And if she can do it—if she can go from hiding behind her office, ready to quit, to running ten thriving practices while also being present for her family—then you can too. But it requires a decision.

The decision to stop surviving and start designing.

The decision to invest in systems, boundaries, and leverage.

The decision to think beyond the chair and build something that lasts.

And that decision starts today.

What This Means for You

Your career does not have to look like anyone else's.

You do not have to work four days a week for 30 years seeing patients back-to-back.

You do not have to choose between being a great dentist and being present for your family.

You do not have to burn out trying to do everything yourself.

You can design something different. Something sustainable. Something that evolves with you.

Block time for business work. Redesign your schedule as your life changes. Build systems and leverage. Think in phases.

And most importantly: **Give yourself permission to evolve.**

You are not the same person you were when you graduated dental school. And you will not be the same person ten years from now.

Your career should grow with you. Not grind you down.

So ask yourself:

- What do I want the next phase of my career to look like?
- What systems do I need to build to make that possible?
- What do I need to let go of?
- What do I need to step into?

And then start building.

One decision at a time. One system at a time. One boundary at a time.

Until you look up one day and realize: **You built a career that lasts.** Not just financially. But physically, mentally, emotionally, and relationally. A career you love. A life you do not want to escape from.

That is what is possible.

And that is what the next chapter is about: the systems that maintain it. The early warning systems that keep you from slipping back into burnout. The practices that make sustainability the default instead of the exception.

Because building something great is one thing. Maintaining it is another.

And that is where we go next.

Reflection Questions:

1. What phase of your career are you in right now? What does the next phase require from you?
2. If you could design your ideal week with no constraints, what would it look like? How different is that from your current schedule?
3. What is one thing you need to let go of (a belief, a responsibility, a way of working) to move into the next phase of your career?
4. Where could you build leverage in your practice? What could you delegate or systematize that would free up your time?
5. What do you want your legacy to be beyond the chair? What are you building that will outlast your clinical career?

PART IV
Maintenance & Scaling

CHAPTER 10

The Early Warning System

Dr. Kalli Hale knows the signs now. The tightness in her chest when she opens her schedule for the week. The increased heart rate.The irritability at home over minor things. The difficulty of falling asleep even though she is exhausted. The urge to check her phone compulsively, scanning for problems.

These are not random symptoms. They are data points. Early warnings that stress is creeping back in. And now, instead of ignoring them or pushing through them, she pays attention.

Because here is what she learned the hard way: **Burnout does not announce itself with a bang. It creeps in quietly, one compromised boundary at a time, one skipped lunch at a time, one "yes" when you should have said "no" at a time.**

And if you do not catch it early, you end up back where you started.

Burnout recovery doesn't mean you prevent stress entirely—stress is unavoidable. But a system that catches stress before it becomes burnout is key. She now has the ability to identify when she is veering off course, so she can correct quickly.

This is maintenance mode. And it is the difference between temporary recovery and lasting transformation.

Because recovering from burnout once is hard. But staying recovered for decades? That requires vigilance.

This chapter is about the early warning system you need to build—the practices, the awareness, the tools—that keep you from slipping back into the patterns that burned you out in the first place.

Maintenance Mode: What to Watch For

Burnout does not happen overnight. And it does not come back overnight either.

You might skip one boundary. If you have added a different line of work outside of clinical dentistry, it is easy to slip into doing too much again. You tolerate one extra thing on your schedule. Then another. Owning multiple dental practices isn't for the faint at heart, and Dr. Kalli has personally experienced what back-to-back zoom calls can do if you don't schedule breaks. And before you know it, you could be slipping into old patterns.

Here is what to watch for:

Physical Red Flags

- Sleep disruption (trouble falling asleep, waking up in the night, waking up exhausted)
- Increased muscle tension (jaw clenching, shoulder tightness, headaches)
- Digestive issues (nausea, loss of appetite, stress eating)
- Fatigue that does not improve with rest
- Getting sick more frequently (colds, infections—signs your immune system is compromised)

Emotional Red Flags

- Irritability or short temper, especially at home
- Feeling numb or detached from patients and work
- Difficulty finding joy in things that used to be enjoyable
- Increased anxiety or sense of dread
- Feeling overwhelmed by tasks that used to be manageable

Behavioral Red Flags

- Skipping breaks or lunches
- Saying yes when you want to say no

- Checking email or messages compulsively
- Working late or taking work home more frequently
- Avoiding difficult but necessary conversations
- Using alcohol, food, or other substances to cope

Relational Red Flags

- Withdrawing from friends or family
- Snapping at your spouse or kids
- Feeling resentful of people who need things from you
- Canceling social plans because you are too tired
- Feeling like no one understands what you are going through

The key is to notice these early. Before they compound. Before they become crisis-level.

Dr. Kalli checks in with herself regularly. She asks: *Am I experiencing any of these symptoms? If so, how many? And for how long? Can I identify the real issue for the feelings I have in this moment?*

One symptom for a few days is normal stress. Multiple symptoms for multiple weeks is a warning sign. And when she sees the warning signs, she acts. Immediately. She does not wait for it to get worse. She does not tell herself she will deal with it later. She recalibrates now. Deep breaths, clear thinking, take a walk, recoup.

Maintenance mode is about early detection and quick response.

Catch it early. Address it quickly. Prevent it from escalating.

The 3Cs Method: Catch, Check, Change

One of the most powerful tools Dr. Kalli uses to maintain her mental health is what she learned from *The Burnout Solution*: the **3Cs Method.**

It is a simple framework for interrupting negative thought patterns before they spiral.

Catch, Check, Change.

Here is how it works:

1. Catch the thought.

The first step is awareness. You cannot change a thought pattern if you do not notice it.

So when you feel yourself getting stressed, anxious, or overwhelmed, pause. Ask: *What am I thinking right now?*

Most of the time, you will catch a catastrophic or negative thought.

This patient is going to be unhappy.

My schedule is impossible.

I can't keep doing this.

Everything is falling apart.

Just notice it. Name it. Bring it into conscious awareness.

Example: Dr. Kalli is looking at her schedule for the week. She feels her chest tighten. She pauses and asks, *What am I thinking?*

The thought: *This schedule is too packed. I'm never going to get through this. I'm going to fall behind and disappoint everyone.*

2. Check the thought.

Once you have caught the thought, ask: **Is this thought accurate?**

Not "Is it possible?" Everything is possible. The question is: *Is this thought based on facts, or is it based on fear and catastrophizing?*

Look for evidence. Challenge the thought.

Is the schedule actually impossible? Or just challenging?

Have I gotten through difficult schedules before?

What evidence do I have that I will disappoint everyone?

Am I catastrophizing or problem-solving?

Most of the time, you will realize: the thought is not accurate. It is an exaggeration. A fear-based prediction. A story you are telling yourself.

Example: Dr. Kalli checks the thought.

Is this schedule actually impossible?

No. It is full, but she has buffer time built in. She has an associate who can help if needed. She has gotten through schedules like this before.

Will I definitely fall behind and disappoint everyone?

No. That is a prediction, not a fact. And even if she runs a little behind, patients will be fine. Her team will handle it.

The thought is catastrophizing. It is not based on reality.

3. Change the thought.

Once you have identified that the thought is inaccurate or unhelpful, replace it with a more accurate, grounding thought.

Not a fake positive affirmation. Not toxic positivity. Just a more realistic, balanced thought.

This schedule is full, but I've handled full schedules before. I have systems in place. I can get through this one day at a time.

If I start to feel overwhelmed, I can take a 15-second reset between patients.

I'm good. This is temporary.

Example: Dr. Kalli changes the thought.

Old thought: *This schedule is too packed. I'm never going to get through this. I'm going to fall behind and disappoint everyone.*

New thought: *This schedule is full, but it's manageable. I've done harder weeks than this. I have my 15-second resets. I have my team. I'm good.*

And just like that, the anxiety decreases. Not completely. But enough that she can move forward instead of spiraling.

The 3Cs Method works because it interrupts the automatic catastrophizing that fuels burnout.

Your brain is wired to scan for threats. And when you are stressed, it starts seeing threats everywhere—even when they do not exist.

The 3Cs Method forces you to slow down, evaluate, and correct.

Catch the thought. Check if it is accurate. Change it to something more helpful.

Do this consistently, and you train your brain to default to realistic thinking instead of catastrophic thinking.

And that is one of the most powerful burnout prevention tools there is.

Tracking Your "What If" Thoughts

Dr. Kalli used to lie awake at night running through worst-case scenarios.

What if the crown doesn't fit?

What if the patient complains?

What if I miss something in the exam?

What if we don't make payroll this month?

What if that employee quits?

Each "what if" triggered another. And by the time she finally fell asleep, her nervous system was in overdrive.

Now, she tracks them.

She keeps a small notebook (or a note on her phone). And when she catches herself spiraling with "what if" thoughts, she writes them down.

Not to obsess over them. But to get them out of her head. And to track patterns.

At the end of the week, she reviews the list. And she asks:

How many of these "what if" thoughts actually came true?

The answer, almost always, is zero. Or maybe one out of twenty.

The crown fit fine. The patient was happy. She did not miss anything. They made payroll. The employee did not quit.

She spent hours of mental energy worrying about things that never happened. She also learned from The Burnout Solution not to let things bother her for longer than it took the incident to occur in the first place!

Tracking your "what if" thoughts does two things:

1. It externalizes the thoughts so they are not swirling in your head.

Writing them down creates distance. They become something you can look at objectively instead of something that feels overwhelming and consuming.

2. It provides data that your brain is catastrophizing.

When you see, week after week, that 95% of your "what if" thoughts never materialize, you start to trust that your brain is being overly dramatic.

And that makes it easier to dismiss the thoughts when they arise.

Oh, there's my brain catastrophizing again. I don't need to engage with this.

Here is the practice:

Keep a "What If" log for 30 days. Every time you catch yourself spiraling with a "what if" thought, write it down.

At the end of the month, go through the list. Mark which ones actually happened.

You will be shocked at how few of them came true.

And that data will help you stop taking every "what if" thought seriously.

Physical Symptoms as Data (Not Weakness)

Dr. Kalli used to ignore her body.

Headaches? Take ibuprofen and keep going.

Stomach issues? Probably just something she ate.

Insomnia? She would catch up on sleep later.

Muscle tension? Everyone has that.

She treated physical symptoms as annoyances to push through. Not as signals that something was wrong.

But her body was trying to tell her something. And when she ignored the whispers, it eventually screamed—186/120.

Now, she listens.

She treats physical symptoms as **data.** Not as weakness. Not as something to be ashamed of. But as information about how her nervous system is responding to stress.

Here is how to use physical symptoms as data:

1. Notice them without judgment.

When you feel tension in your shoulders, or your stomach is upset, or you cannot sleep—do not berate yourself. Do not tell yourself you are weak or broken.

Just notice. *My body is giving me information.*

2. Ask: What is my body trying to tell me?

Physical symptoms are often your nervous system's way of saying: *Something is off. You are pushing too hard. You need to slow down.*

Headaches might be saying: *You are clenching your jaw. You are tense.*

Digestive issues might be saying: *You are in chronic stress. Your nervous system is in fight-or-flight.*

Insomnia might be saying: *Your mind is racing. You are not winding down properly.*

3. Respond with care, not with punishment.

Do not ignore the symptoms. Do not just medicate them and keep going.

Respond. Take a break. Do some deep breathing. Go for a walk. Stretch. Journal. Talk to someone.

Give your body what it needs instead of demanding that it keep performing despite the warning signs.

Dr. Kalli now keeps a blood pressure cuff in her office. Not because she has hypertension. But because it gives her objective data.

If she feels off, she checks her blood pressure. If it is elevated, she knows: *My body is stressed. I need to do something about this. Now.*

And she does. She takes a walk. She does breathing exercises. She cancels something non-essential. She enforces a boundary.

Your body is not your enemy. It is your early warning system.

Listen to it.

Quarterly Practice Audits

Dr. Kalli schedules a **quarterly practice audit** every three months.

This is dedicated time—usually a half day—where she steps back and evaluates how things are going.

Not just financially. But holistically.

She asks:

Clinically:

- Am I still enjoying the cases I am seeing?
- Are there procedures I am doing that drain me?
- Am I staying current with CE and skills development?

Operationally:

- Are the systems working, or are there bottlenecks?
- Is the team functioning well, or is there dysfunction?
- Are patients having a great experience, or are there complaints?

Financially:

- Are we hitting our targets?

- Are there expenses we could reduce?
- Are we collecting well, or is AR piling up?

Personally:

- Am I maintaining my boundaries?
- Am I taking time off?
- Am I experiencing any burnout symptoms?

Team:

- Is anyone struggling or showing signs of burnout?
- Do we need to hire additional help?
- Are there training needs?

She does not do this alone. She involves her executive team and her husband Dr. Kyle (who is the COO of the business). For you, it may be you and your office manager.

And she uses the audit to make adjustments **before small problems become big problems.**

Maybe she notices she is taking on too many difficult cases and needs to delegate some to associates. Or maybe she sees stress in her office manager that needs to be acknowledged.

Maybe she sees that the front desk is getting overwhelmed and needs to hire another person.

Maybe she realizes she has been skipping her Tuesday off too often and needs to recommit to the boundary.

The quarterly audit is preventive maintenance.

It keeps small issues from becoming crises. It keeps you from drifting off course without realizing it.

And it ensures that you are proactively managing your practice and your life instead of just reacting to whatever comes up.

Block time every quarter to step back and evaluate. You cannot fix what you do not see. And you cannot see clearly if you never stop long enough to look.

Block time off weekly to get in sync with yourself, your goals, and your growth.

Regular Check-Ins With Yourself

In addition to quarterly audits, Dr. Kalli does **weekly check-ins with herself.**

Every Tuesday morning during her blocked off time, she sits down with a journal and asks:

1. How am I feeling physically, mentally, and emotionally?

She rates herself on a scale of 1-10 in each area. If any area is below a 7, she asks: *What is contributing to this? What do I need to change this week?*

2. What went well this week?

She writes down wins, moments of joy, things she is proud of. This counteracts the brain's negativity bias and helps her see the good instead of only focusing on problems.

3. What did not go well this week?

She names the challenges, the frustrations, the things that did not work. Not to dwell on them, but to identify patterns and make adjustments.

4. What professional goals do I have right now?

Something tangible to achieve in the coming 6 months

5. What personal goals do I have right now??

Maybe it is scheduling a massage. Maybe it is scheduling a date night with her husband. Maybe it is having a difficult conversation she has been avoiding.

She picks one thing and commits to it.

This weekly check-in takes 10-15 minutes. But it keeps her grounded.

It prevents her from going weeks or months without noticing that stress is building. It keeps her connected to herself instead of just running on autopilot.

Create a regular rhythm for checking in with yourself. Weekly. Bi-weekly. Whatever works.

But do it consistently. Because you cannot course-correct if you do not know you are off course.

Transition Rituals: Clocking Out Mentally

One of Dr. Kalli's biggest struggles was leaving work at work.

She would finish her day, drive home, and her mind would still be at the office. Replaying cases. Worrying about patients. Planning for tomorrow. Bringing things up at home with Dr. Kyle.

She was physically home, but mentally still working.

And that meant she never truly recovered. Her nervous system never got a break.

So she built **transition rituals.** Small practices that signal to her brain: *The workday is over. You can let go now.*

Here is what she does:

1. The 5-minute debrief.

Before she ends her work day, she takes five minutes to write down anything she needs to remember for tomorrow. Tasks to complete. Patients to follow up with. Decisions to make.

Getting it out of her head and onto paper means she does not have to hold it in her mental RAM all night.

2. The physical transition.

She changes clothes when she gets home. Work clothes come off. Comfortable clothes go on.

This signals to her brain: *You are not at work anymore. You are home.*

3. The mental separation.

On her drive home, she does a breathing exercise (box breathing). Or listens to music. Or calls a friend.

Something that occupies her mind so she is not replaying the day.

Then she gets out of the car and focuses on being present with her family.

Why this matters:

If you do not have a transition ritual, work bleeds into home. You are physically there, but mentally absent.

And that is exhausting for you and unfair to your family.

Create a transition ritual. It does not have to be elaborate. Just something consistent that signals to your brain: *Work is over. Recovery begins now.*

Self-Care That Actually Works for Dentists

Let's talk about self-care.

Not the Instagram version. Not bubble baths and face masks (though those are fine if they work for you).

But actual, functional self-care that prevents burnout for dentists.

Here is what does not work:

- Generic advice to "just relax" or "take a vacation" (if the systems are broken, a vacation is just a delay before you come back to the same chaos)

- Self-care that requires you to add more to your schedule (you are already overwhelmed—adding a yoga class you do not have time for is not helpful)
- Self-care that ignores the root causes (if your boundaries are the problem, a massage is not the solution)

Here is what does work:

1. Boundary enforcement.

The most important form of self-care is protecting your time, energy, and capacity. Saying no when you need to say no. Blocking off time for yourself. Not being available 24/7.

2. Physical movement that you enjoy.

Exercise doesn't have to be something you force yourself to do and suffer through. It can be movement that feels good. Walking. Stretching. Dancing. Playing with your kids.

Movement that regulates your nervous system and gets you out of your head.

3. Connection with people who refuel you.

Time with friends who make you laugh. Conversations with people who get it. Relationships that give you energy instead of draining it.

4. Activities that create flow.

Hobbies. Creative pursuits. Anything that gets you into a state of flow where you lose track of time and your mind is fully engaged in something other than dentistry.

For Dr. Kalli, it is playing the piano or cooking. For you, it might be sewing, or gardening, or exercising.

5. Sleep.

Non-negotiable. If you are not sleeping, nothing else works. Protect your sleep like your life depends on it. Because it does.

Self-care is not an indulgence. It is maintenance.

You do not skip oil changes on your car because you are too busy. You do not skip charging your phone because you do not have time.

Your body and mind are no different. They require maintenance.

Build self-care into your systems. Make it non-negotiable.

When to Get Help (Therapy vs. Coaching vs. Mentorship)

Dr. Kalli gets asked this all the time: *When do I need professional help? And what kind?*

Here is how she thinks about it:

Therapy is for when you are dealing with significant mental health issues—depression, anxiety, trauma, relational dysfunction.

If you are having intrusive thoughts, if you cannot function, if your relationships are falling apart, if you are using substances to cope—you need therapy.

Therapy helps you process the past, understand your patterns, and heal what is broken.

Coaching is for when you are functional but stuck. You know what you want, but you do not know how to get there. Or you keep sabotaging yourself and you need accountability and strategy.

Coaching is forward-focused. It is about setting goals and building the skills and systems to achieve them.

Dr. Kalli worked through *The Burnout Solution* like a coaching program. It gave her tools, frameworks, and practices to change her thinking and her behavior. Other dentists coached with Dr. Sharon to overcome their burnout more quickly and with more support.

Mentorship is for when you need guidance from someone who has been where you want to go.

Dr. Kalli mentors other dentists on practice management, airway cases, and burnout prevention. She does not provide therapy. She provides practical advice based on her experience.

Mentorship is about learning from someone who has already walked the path.

How to decide:

If you are in crisis, start with therapy. Get stabilized.

If you are functional but struggling to make changes, consider coaching.

If you have specific professional challenges, find a mentor who has solved those challenges.

And often, you need more than one. Dr. Kalli has worked with therapists, coaches, and mentors at different points in her journey.

Do not wait until you are in crisis to get help. Preventive support is always easier than crisis intervention.

And there is no shame in asking for help. The strongest people are the ones who know when they need support.

Your Personal Go-To Tools List

Dr. Kalli has a list of tools, practices, and reminders that she can reference when she feels stress creeping back in.

Because when you are stressed, you cannot think clearly. You forget what helps. You revert to old patterns.

But if you have a pre-made list, you can just open it and pick something.

Here is what is on Dr. Kalli's list:

- something fun to look forward to
- Ask Take three deep breaths
- Do the 15-second reset
- Use the 3Cs Method (Catch, Check, Change)
- Check my blood pressure

- Go for a 10-minute walk
- Call Dr. Kyle or my parents
- Read a chapter from *The Burnout Solution*
- Journal for 5 minutes
- Enforce one boundary I have been letting slip
- Say "I'm good" and "It's temporary"
- Review my "What If" log to remind myself most of my fears do not come true
- Schedule for help

She does not use all of these every time. She just picks the one or two that feel most relevant in the moment.

Create your own go-to tools list.

Write down the practices, reminders, and strategies that help you. The things you have learned. The tools that work.

And when you are struggling, open the list. Pick one thing. Do it.

Every week during her administrative time, Dr. Kalli sits down and has what she calls her personal synchro time. In her journal, she answers the following three questions:

1. List 3 successes from last week
2. What are next week's goals?
3. What are your big-picture goals for the next year and beyond that belong on my vision board?

You do not have to fix everything. You just have to take one small step toward recalibration.

What This All Means

Recovering from burnout is hard.

But staying recovered? That is the real work.

Because life does not stop. Stress does not stop. New challenges arise. Old patterns try to creep back in.

And if you do not have an early warning system—if you do not have practices in place to catch stress before it becomes burnout—you will find yourself right back where you started.

The early warning system is not about perfection. It is about awareness and responsiveness.

You notice the signs. You check in with yourself regularly. You use the tools. You course-correct quickly.

And when you do that consistently, burnout becomes something you prevent instead of something you recover from over and over again.

Dr. Kalli still has hard weeks. She still feels stressed sometimes. She still has moments where she thinks, "*Man, I'm juggling a lot!*"

But she does not spiral. She does not let it compound. She catches it early and recalibrates. And that is the difference between someone who burns out repeatedly and someone who builds a sustainable career.

Build your early warning system. Maintain it. Trust it.

Because the goal is not just to survive this year. The goal is to thrive for the next 30 years. And that requires vigilance. But it is worth it.

Reflection Questions:

1. What are your personal early warning signs that stress is building? (Physical, emotional, behavioral, relational)
2. When was the last time you did a thorough check-in with yourself? What would you discover if you did one this week?

3. What is one transition ritual you could create to help you mentally "clock out" from work?
4. What tools or practices help you when you are struggling? Could you create a go-to list?
5. Do you need professional help right now? (Therapy, coaching, mentorship) If so, what is stopping you from reaching out?

CHAPTER 11

From Exhausted To Extraordinary

Dr. Kalli Hale will never forget the moment she realized she had made it to the other side.

She was driving to pick up her kids from school. It was a Tuesday afternoon—her day off from clinical work. She had just finished a mentorship call with a dentist in California who was on the edge of burnout, struggling with the same things she had struggled with years ago.

And as she drove, she felt something she had not felt in years: **peace.** Not the absence of stress. She still had a full schedule. She still had many practices to oversee. She still had challenges and problems to solve.

But she was not drowning. She was not white-knuckling her way through the day. She was not fantasizing about her practice burning down so she would have an excuse to quit. She was present. Engaged. Alive. And she thought: *I love my life. I actually love what I do.*

This was not where she thought she would end up when she stood behind her dental office, ready to walk away from everything. She thought burnout meant the end of her dental career. That the only way out was to quit. But what she discovered was something far more powerful: **Burnout was not the end. It was the catalyst for transformation.**

The journey from exhausted to extraordinary is not about working harder or achieving more. It is about becoming someone different in the process.

Someone with boundaries. Someone who knows their worth is not tied to their productivity. Someone who can lead without sacrificing themselves. Someone who designs their life instead of surviving it.

This final chapter is about what is possible on the other side of burnout. Not just surviving. Not just recovering. But thriving in ways you cannot imagine when you are in the thick of it.

The Real Reward: Who You Become in the Process

When Dr. Kalli started working through *The Burnout Solution*, she wanted relief.

She wanted to stop feeling anxious all the time. She wanted to sleep through the night. She wanted to stop having panic attacks about her schedule. She really wanted herself back.

Relief was the goal. Get back to baseline. Get back to "fine."

But what she got was so much more than relief. She got transformation.

The work of recovering from burnout forced her to confront things she had been avoiding her whole life:

Her perfectionism. The relentless belief that she had to be flawless to be worthy. That every mistake was a character indictment. That anything less than perfect was failure.

She had to learn: *Excellent is enough. Good enough is actually good enough. My worth as a human being is not determined by my performance.*

Her people-pleasing. The inability to say no. The belief that disappointing someone meant she was a bad person. The compulsion to make everyone happy at her own expense.

She had to learn: *I cannot serve everyone. Boundaries are not selfish. Saying no to some people allows me to say yes to the right people.*

Her control issues. The belief that if she did not do everything herself, it would not get done right. The inability to trust others. The need to micromanage every detail.

She had to learn: *I can delegate without losing quality. Empowering others is leadership. I cannot scale by doing everything myself.*

Her fusion with her work. The belief that her identity was inseparable from being a dentist. That her worth came from her productivity. That she was nothing outside of her career.

She had to learn: *I am a human being with inherent worth. My work is valuable, but it is not what makes me valuable. I exist beyond the chair.*

These shifts were painful. Uncomfortable. Difficult.

But they made her a better dentist, a better leader, a better spouse, a better parent, and a better human.

And that is the real reward.

Not just a better schedule. Not just less stress. But becoming someone who can handle stress differently. Someone who can lead without burning out. Someone who can build something extraordinary without sacrificing everything else.

The journey from exhausted to extraordinary is not about fixing your circumstances. It is about transforming yourself.

And when you transform yourself, your circumstances change as a byproduct. *Remember, you get what you tolerate.*

From Victim of the Schedule to CEO of Yourself

There is a fundamental shift that happens when you recover from burnout.

You stop seeing yourself as a victim of your circumstances and start seeing yourself as the CEO of your life.

When you are burned out, you feel powerless.

Your schedule controls you. Your patients control you. Your staff controls you. Insurance controls you. Debt controls you.

You are a passenger in your own life, reacting to what comes at you, while trying to make a living.

But recovery is about reclaiming power.

Not power over others. But power over yourself. Your choices. Your time. Your energy.

Dr. Kalli describes this shift: "I went from thinking, 'I have to do this' to thinking, 'I get to do this.'"

That small reframe changed everything.

I have to see this patient becomes *I get to help this patient, because they align with my ideal patient avatar.*

I have to stay late becomes *I choose to protect my boundary and leave at 3 p.m.*

I have to answer this message becomes *I choose when and how I engage with patient communications.*

When you shift from "I have to" to "I choose," you reclaim agency. You are no longer a victim of your schedule. You are the designer of your schedule. You are no longer controlled by external demands. You evaluate those demands and decide which ones you will meet. You are no longer at the mercy of other people's expectations. You set your own standards and boundaries.

This is what it means to be the CEO of yourself.

You take full responsibility for your life. Not in a punishing way. But in an empowering way.

You stop blaming circumstances and start asking: *What can I do differently? What is within my control? How can I design this better?*

And when you live from that place, everything changes. You stop feeling helpless. You stop feeling trapped. You stop feeling like burnout is inevitable. Because you are making active choices instead of passively reacting.

The shift from victim to CEO is the shift from exhausted to extraordinary.

What's Possible Beyond Survival

When you are in the thick of burnout, survival is the only goal.

Just get through today. Just make it to the weekend. Just survive until things calm down.

But things never calm down. Not on their own. And survival is exhausting.

Dr. Kalli spent years in survival mode. An uncomfortable place to be which affected every aspect of her life.But once she rebuilt—once she set boundaries, built systems, hired help, reclaimed her mental health—she realized something:

Survival was not the way to live your life. Thriving was.

And thriving opened up possibilities she had never considered. She did not just want to see patients and go home. She wanted to build something bigger. She wanted to train other dentists. She wanted to open multiple practices. She wanted to create new models of care. She wanted to mentor people going through what she went through. And once she was no longer drowning, she had the capacity to do it.

Here is what becomes possible when you move beyond survival:

You can explore new models of care.

You can become a mentor and thought leader.

You can build multiple income streams.

You can design a life that integrates work and family.

You can leave a legacy.

Teledentistry, Mentorship, and Models You Haven't Considered

One of the most limiting beliefs dentists have is: **The only way to make money as a dentist is to see patients in a chair.** And that belief keeps people trapped. Because if that is the only option, then you can never truly scale. You can never step back. You are always dependent on trading time for money. But Dr. Kalli discovered: there are so many other ways to add value as a dentist.

Teledentistry

Dr. Kalli's teledentistry company provides virtual consultations and care coordination for underserved populations.

She is not doing clinical work herself. She is overseeing a team of providers. She is building systems. She is creating access for people who would not otherwise get care. And it is scalable. It is not dependent on her being in one place at one time.

Group practice ownership with associate dentists

Dr. Kalli now has ten locations with associate dentists producing in each one. This is leverage. This is how you scale beyond your own capacity.

Consulting and practice management

Dentists who have built successful practices can consult with others who are struggling. You are paid for your knowledge and experience, not your hands-on clinical time.

Speaking and education

Conferences. Webinars. Podcasts. Online courses. If you have expertise, you can teach it. And teaching scales in ways clinical work does not.

Mentorship programs

Dr. Kalli runs a mentorship program for dentists who want to build airway-focused practices. She is paid for her guidance, not her clinical work.

Product development or partnerships

Some dentists create products—instruments, materials, software—and earn royalties.

Others partner with companies as advisors or consultants.

The point is: clinical dentistry is not the only option.

And the more income streams you have, the more freedom you have. You can work clinically because you love it, not because you have to. And that changes everything.

Building a Practice You Don't Want to Escape From

Dr. Kalli used to fantasize about her practice burning down. Not because she hated dentistry. But because she felt trapped. And destruction felt like the only way out.

Now, she loves her practices. Plural.

Not because they are perfect. Not because there are no challenges. But because she designed them intentionally to support the life she wants.

Here is what makes a practice sustainable instead of suffocating:

1. It is built around your values, not just production.

Dr. Kalli's practices focus on airway, sleep, and whole-body health. That is what lights her up. That is the work she loves.

She is not trying to be everything to everyone. She is serving her ideal patients with the care she is passionate about.

2. It has systems that create predictability.

The patient experience framework. The training protocols. The handoff systems.

Everything runs smoothly because there are systems. Not chaos masked as productivity.

3. It has a team you trust.

Dr. Kalli has built teams that can run the practices without her being there every day.

She can step back because she trusts them. And that trust is built on training, clear expectations, and ongoing communication.

4. It has boundaries that protect you.

Dr. Kalli does not see patients after 3 p.m. She does not work on Tuesdays (clinical work). She does not answer patient messages after hours.

The practice respects her boundaries. And that makes it sustainable.

5. It generates income beyond your clinical time.

Associate dentists. Multiple locations. Other revenue streams.

Dr. Kalli's income is not entirely dependent on how many hours she spends in the operatory.

When you build a practice this way, you do not want to escape from it.

You want to grow it. Improve it. Share it. Because it is not draining you. It is energizing you.

The Legacy Question: What Do You Want to Leave Behind?

Dr. Kalli is in her 30s. She has decades of career left. But she is already thinking about legacy.

What do I want to leave behind?

Not just financially. But relationally, professionally, and in terms of impact.

She wants to have trained a generation of dentists who practice differently.

Dentists who do not burn out. Dentists who design sustainable practices. Dentists who deliver excellent care without sacrificing their families or their health.

She wants to have created models of care that improve access.

The teledentistry company. The group practice model. Systems that make great dental care available to people who would not otherwise have it.

She wants her kids to experience her as present.

Not perfect. But present. Not someone who was always at work. But someone who showed up for them.

She wants to have built something that outlasts her clinical career.

Practices that will thrive long after she stops seeing patients. Systems that will be used by others. Knowledge that will be passed on.

Legacy is not about being famous. It is about being intentional.

What are you building that will outlast you?

What impact do you want to have beyond the chair?

What do you want people to say about you when you are gone?

These are not questions to answer in your 60s. These are questions to answer now.

Because the legacy you leave is built day by day, choice by choice, over decades.

And if you do not think about it intentionally, you will default to whatever happens.

Think about your legacy. And then build toward it.

Hope for Those Reading in the Thick of It

If you are reading this and you are in the thick of burnout right now—if you are drowning, if you are barely holding it together, if you are one bad day away from quitting—hear this:

You are not broken. Stick with it.

You are not weak. There is relief once you fix the issue.

You are not failing. But you will if your mind can't escape fight or flight.

You are in a system that was never designed to be sustainable. And you are carrying more than any one person should carry.

But here is the hope:

It does not have to stay this way.

Dr. Kalli changed how she thought. She set boundaries. She built systems. She hired help. She designed differently.

And you can too.

It will not be easy. Change is hard. Boundaries are uncomfortable. Building systems takes time.

But it is possible. And it is worth it. Because the alternative—continuing to burn out, continuing to sacrifice, continuing to survive instead of thrive—is unsustainable.

You will not make it 30 years at this pace. Your body will not allow it. Your mind will not allow it. Your relationships will not allow it.

So the question is not *if* you will change. The question is *when.* And the sooner you start, the sooner you get to the other side.

Start small.

Pick one thing from this book. One boundary. One system. One mindset shift.

Do that one thing this week. And then do the next thing next week.

You do not have to fix everything at once. You just have to take the first step. And before you know it, you will look up and realize: you are not drowning anymore. You are breathing. You are designing. You are thriving.

The journey from exhausted to extraordinary is not about working harder.

It is about working smarter. Thinking differently. Building intentionally. And it is available to you. Right now. Today. **You just have to decide.**

Are you going to keep surviving? Or are you going to start designing? The choice is yours.

Bonus Resources

Burnout recovery doesn't happen by just reading about it; it happens by changing your day-to-day practice patterns. To help you implement the strategies in this book, we have created a suite of practical, printable tools designed specifically for busy dental professionals.

1. The Dental Burnout Spectrum Self-Assessment

A printable burnout screening tool based on the framework in Chapter 1. Use it to identify early warning signs, track progress, and start meaningful conversations with colleagues and team members.

2. The What If Thought Log

Download the 30-Day "What If" Thought Log and test your predictions against reality. Most dentists are shocked by how many feared outcomes never happen.

3. The Handoff Sheet Template

A plug-and-play communication tool designed to eliminate practice bottlenecks and operational friction. Use it to align your team, clarify clinical responsibilities, and ensure seamless patient transitions between the front office and clinical staff.

4. The Patient First SleepWell Framework

A step-by-step clinical and behavioral workflow for integrating dental sleep medicine into your practice without burning out your team. This framework helps you confidently identify airway issues, communicate value to patients, and protect your own time.

5. The Go-To Tools List Template

A fillable personal toolkit card based on the early warning system in Chapter 10. Pre-program your favorite nervous system regulation strategies, grounding mantras, and non-negotiable boundaries so you can bypass decision fatigue and ground yourself instantly when acute stress strikes.

Download the complete toolkit at: www.dentalburnoutsolution.com

What Comes Next

This is not the end of the journey. It is the beginning. Because recovering from burnout is not a destination. It is a practice. You will have hard weeks. You will slip back into old patterns occasionally. You will face new challenges.

But you will have tools. You will have systems. You will have awareness. And most importantly, you will have proof that change is possible. Because you did it once. And you can do it again.

Dr. Kalli still has hard days. But they do not define her anymore. They do not derail her. Because she has built something sustainable. Something resilient. Something extraordinary. And so can you.

This book is your roadmap. The diagnosis. The stabilization. The root causes. The systems. The team-building. The career design. The early warning system.

Everything you need is here. Now it is up to you to implement it.

You have everything you need to go from exhausted to extraordinary.

You just have to decide you are worth it. And you are. You absolutely are.

Final Reflection Questions:

1. Who have you become through your struggles with burnout? What strengths have you discovered in yourself?
2. What would it look like for you to shift from victim of your circumstances to CEO of your life?
3. What is one model of dentistry (teledentistry, mentorship, group practice, etc.) that you have not considered but might explore?
4. If you were designing your ideal work-life integration with no constraints, what would it look like?
5. What do you want your legacy to be? And what is one thing you can do this week to start building toward it?
6. What is the very first step you will take after finishing this book? (Be specific. Name it. Commit to it.)

A Final Word

This book is the story of one dentist who was burned out to the point of wanting to throw it all away. But she recovered and rebuilt her practice and life in a sustainable way.

And now, through this book, we are passing the blueprint to you.

Use it. Implement it. Adapt it to your situation. And then, when you make it to the other side, pass it on. Because the dental profession needs more people who refuse to burn out. Be one of those people.

The profession needs you. Your patients need you. Your family needs you. And you need you—whole, healthy, and thriving.

Go build something extraordinary.

THE INVITATION

Join The Movement

This book is not just about Dr. Kalli's story.It is not just about your individual recovery from burnout.

It is about a movement.

A movement of dentists who refuse to accept that burnout is inevitable. Who refuse to sacrifice their health, their families, and their joy for their careers.

A movement of dentists who are building differently. Who are setting boundaries. Who are creating systems. Who are prioritizing sustainability over constant growth.

A movement of dentists who are proving that you can be excellent without being exhausted. That you can build something extraordinary without burning out.

Dr. Kalli is not the only one.

There are dentists all over the world who have made this shift. Who have gone from exhausted to extraordinary.

And when you join them—when you do the work, implement the tools, build the systems—you become part of something bigger.

You become proof that change is possible.

This is the invitation: Join the movement.

Not by doing more. But by doing differently.

Read this book. Implement the tools. Share what you learn.

Support other dentists who are struggling. Normalize talking about burnout. Create space for people to acknowledge they are not okay. Build practices that do not burn people out—not just you, but your associates, your staff, everyone. And when you make it to the other side, reach back and help someone else across.

Resources for Your Journey:

For more information about Dr. Kalli Hale's mentorship programs and speaking, visit www.thesleepwelljourney.com. She can also be found on instagram @theairwaycentereddentist. We're always looking for passionate dentists to join our team. Visit www.theairwaydentists.com.

For Dr. Sharon Grossman's burnout recovery coaching program, visit https://drsharongrossman.com/burnoutprogram/.

The Burnout Solution: 7 Steps from Exhausted to Extraordinary by Dr. Sharon Grossman is available wherever books are sold.

One More Thing Before You Go

If this book helped you, do something that takes two minutes and costs nothing: leave a review on Amazon.

Not for us. For the dentist who is Googling "burnout" at midnight, wondering if anyone else feels the way they feel. Your honest words could be the thing that convinces them to pick up this book instead of walking out the back door.

Every review is a hand extended to someone who needs it.

And if you know a dentist who is struggling, silently pushing through, or just "fine" in that way that means anything but, send them this book. You do not have to have a conversation about it. Just put it in their hands. Sometimes the most powerful thing you can do for someone is let them know they are not alone.

The dental profession does not have to keep burning people out. But that changes one dentist at a time. Starting with you.

Just go to http://bit.ly/dentalburnout and scroll down to the bottom left. It looks like this:

Review this product

Share your thoughts with other customers

Write a customer review

Bring This Conversation to Your Conference

If you are organizing a dental conference, study club, or professional development event and want your attendees to leave with tools they can use the next morning, Dr. Sharon Grossman is available as a keynote speaker and continuing education presenter. Her programs on burnout prevention and recovery, leadership, staff retention, and workplace culture are evidence-based, practical, and built for dental audiences. CE credit is available for applicable presentations.

To inquire about availability and topics, visit https://drsharongrossman.com or schedule a call at https://drsharongrossman.com/bookme.

Acknowledgments

By Dr. Kalli Hale

This book was born from one of the most difficult seasons of my life, and it wouldn't exist without the people who stood beside me when I could barely stand on my own.

To my husband, Kyle, you are my rock. When burnout consumed me and I didn't know who I was anymore, you never wavered. You held our world together when I couldn't, and you never once made me feel like I was too much. Thank you for always fixing my problems. I love you more than I can put into words.

To my parents, Jay and Tracy Elliott: thank you for raising me to know I could get back up, no matter how hard I fell. To never quit, to always work hard and eliminate excuses. Your love and support carried me through the darkest days, and your belief in me never faltered. Thank you for setting me up for success at every opportunity! Because of your guidance I am living the life of my dreams.

To my sisters, Jackie and Chelsea: thank you for putting up with me. From the stressed out calls, the tears, the frustration, and every moment in between. I don't know what I would've done without you two! Nothing compares to being able to call your sister and get honest advice from people who truly understand who you are. I love you both!

To Mekenzie Shulse : thank you for helping me raise my babies when I was figuring out how to manage my professional life. Full stop, I couldn't have done this without you. You were there from the beginning of me learning to be a mom, a business owner, and an airway dentist. I am forever grateful for you.

To my associate doctors at The Airway Dentists: this book was written so you never have to go through what I did. You are the reason I turned my pain into a purpose. I hope these pages give you the awareness, the permission, and the tools to protect yourselves before burnout ever takes hold. I will always be there for each of you and hope to leave a memorable place in your heart.

Finally, to my team at New Teeth Dental: you were in the trenches with me every single day during the hardest season of my career. I know I wasn't always easy to work alongside, and yet you stayed. Your loyalty and love carried me through. Without New Teeth Dental, The Airway Dentists wouldn't exist - and for that, I dedicate this book to you.

By Dr. Sharon Grossman

When I wrote *The Burnout Solution* in 2018, I spent two years putting everything I knew onto the page. I wrote it for someone I had not met yet. That is always the leap of faith a writer takes. You do the work, you send it out into the world, and you hope it lands in the right hands.

Dr. Kalli Hale was the right hands.

She did not just read my book. She worked it. Every Tuesday she blocked off for herself, every exercise she completed between patients, every highlight and dog-eared page. She was, in the truest sense, a good student. And it was that faithfulness to the process, in the middle of a real practice with real pressure and real stakes, that planted the seed for everything you are holding right now.

Kalli, you took a framework built in a therapy room and proved it worked in an operatory. You then turned around and championed this work to every dentist in your orbit, because that is who you are. You did not recover quietly. You reached back. I am flattered that my work found you. I am honored that you trusted it enough to build on it.

This collaboration reminded me why I wrote the first book in the first place.

I also want to thank the clients who have trusted me over the years with their most honest moments. The business leaders, founders, and executives who sat across from me and said, out loud, that they were not okay. Coaching is a privilege I do not take lightly. Watching the material I spent years developing actually transform someone's life, in real time, is the reason this work continues. You showed me what was possible. This book exists because of what I learned alongside you.

To every dentist who picks up this book at midnight, exhausted and searching: you are who I wrote it for.

I hope it finds you exactly when you need it.

www.ingramcontent.com/pod-product-compliance
Lightning Source LLC
LaVergne TN
LVHW022037200926
848481LV00003B/710
* 9 7 8 1 9 5 2 4 3 7 0 8 3 *